Lead Contamination

Other titles in the *Emerging Issues in Public Health* series include:

Cell Phone Addiction
Childhood Trauma
Gun Violence
The Opioid Crisis

EMERGING ISSUES IN PUBLIC HEALTH

Lead Contamination

Peggy J. Parks

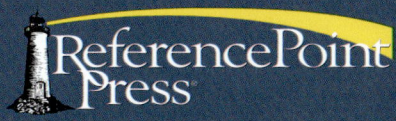

San Diego, CA

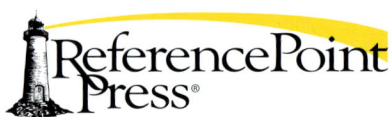

© 2020 ReferencePoint Press, Inc.
Printed in the United States

For more information, contact:
ReferencePoint Press, Inc.
PO Box 27779
San Diego, CA 92198
www.ReferencePointPress.com

ALL RIGHTS RESERVED.
No part of this work covered by the copyright hereon may be reproduced or used in any form or by any means—graphic, electronic, or mechanical, including photocopying, recording, taping, web distribution, or information storage retrieval systems—without the written permission of the publisher.

LIBRARY OF CONGRESS CATALOGING-IN-PUBLICATION DATA

Name: Parks, Peggy J., 1951– author.
Title: Lead Contamination/by Peggy J. Parks.
Description: San Diego, CA: ReferencePoint Press, Inc., 2020. | Series:
  Emerging Issues in Public Health | Audience: Grade 9 to 12. | Includes
  bibliographical references and index.
Identifiers: LCCN 2018060657 (print) | LCCN 2018061614 (ebook) | ISBN
  9781682826720 (eBook) | ISBN 9781682826713 (hardback)
Subjects: LCSH: Lead poisoning—United States.
Classification: LCC RA1231.L4 (ebook) | LCC RA1231.L4 P37 2020 (print) | DDC
  615.9/25688—dc23
LC record available at https://lccn.loc.gov/2018060657

CONTENTS

Introduction   6
Dangerous Metal

Chapter One   10
Public Health Crises in the Making

Chapter Two   23
A Heavy Toll on Human Health

Chapter Three   36
No End in Sight

Chapter Four   49
An Urgent Search for Solutions

Source Notes   63
Organizations and Websites   68
For Further Research   71
Index   73
Picture Credits   79
About the Author   80

INTRODUCTION

Dangerous Metal

Pediatrician Mona Hanna-Attisha of Flint, Michigan, feared for her young patients. Blood tests showed that from 2013 to 2015, the number of Flint children with elevated blood lead levels climbed from 2.4 percent to 4.9 percent, and in high-risk neighborhoods the increase was even greater. Hanna-Attisha knew how dangerous this was; lead is a powerful neurotoxin—meaning a poisonous substance that can cause lasting damage to the brain and other parts of the nervous system. The situation was dire, as she explains: "I could see it in the blood of kids who visited my medical clinic here. . . . Children were being poisoned."[1]

At the same time, residents of Flint had begun noticing changes in the water flowing out of their faucets. It had a strange color, tasted bad, and smelled like rotten eggs. Many complained to the city but got no response, nor did they hear back from state government representatives. When Hanna-Attisha raised the alarm, city and state government officials ridiculed her, attempted to discredit her research, and accused her of trying to cause public hysteria by distorting facts. But she refused to be bullied and would not back down.

In September 2015 Hanna-Attisha held a press conference to release her findings. Her records clearly showed that children's blood lead levels spiked after the city switched its water source, which confirmed what had caused the lead in their bloodstreams. Largely because of her efforts, along with the resulting outrage and widespread publicity, officials in Genesee County, where Flint is located, declared a public health emergency on October 1. The following January President Barack Obama declared a federal emergency in Flint, which freed up millions of dollars in federal aid to assist with the public health crisis.

A Centuries-Old Problem

The Flint water crisis brought new attention to a very old problem—one that was identified centuries ago. Lead, which exists naturally in the earth's crust, was one of the first metals discovered by humans. The potential hazards associated with it were identified as early as 15 BCE, when the Roman architect and civil engineer Marcus Vitruvius found that water could be contaminated when it flowed through lead pipes. "Water is much more wholesome from earthenware pipes than from lead pipes," Vitruvius wrote. "For [water] seems to be made injurious by lead."[2] Over the years and decades and centuries that followed, innumerable other writings warned about the dangers of lead, but that did nothing to curtail its use. Convinced that lead's great value outweighed any potential health risks, scientists continued to develop products with lead that they believed would benefit society.

One of those products was paint. Beginning in the late 1800s, lead-based paint was widely used in the United States. It was preferred to other kinds of paint for many reasons, including durability, washability, and lustrous appearance. In 1921 another lead-based product was created by a General Motors engineer named Thomas Midgley Jr. A heavy, oily form of the metal known as tetraethyl lead was added to gasoline to make motor vehicle engines run more efficiently, with reduced knocking noise. Lead was used to make batteries, water supply pipes, and solder for plumbing, as well as to make fine lead crystal and other glassware, stained glass windows, and other household objects. "We poisoned ourselves with lead during the 20th century in most industrial nations," says radiation science expert Fiona E. McNeill. "We used the metal widely, because lead paint is durable, engines run better on leaded gasoline, and lead water pipes don't rust."[3]

> "We poisoned ourselves with lead during the 20th century in most industrial nations."[3]
>
> —Fiona E. McNeill, a radiation science expert from Hamilton, Canada

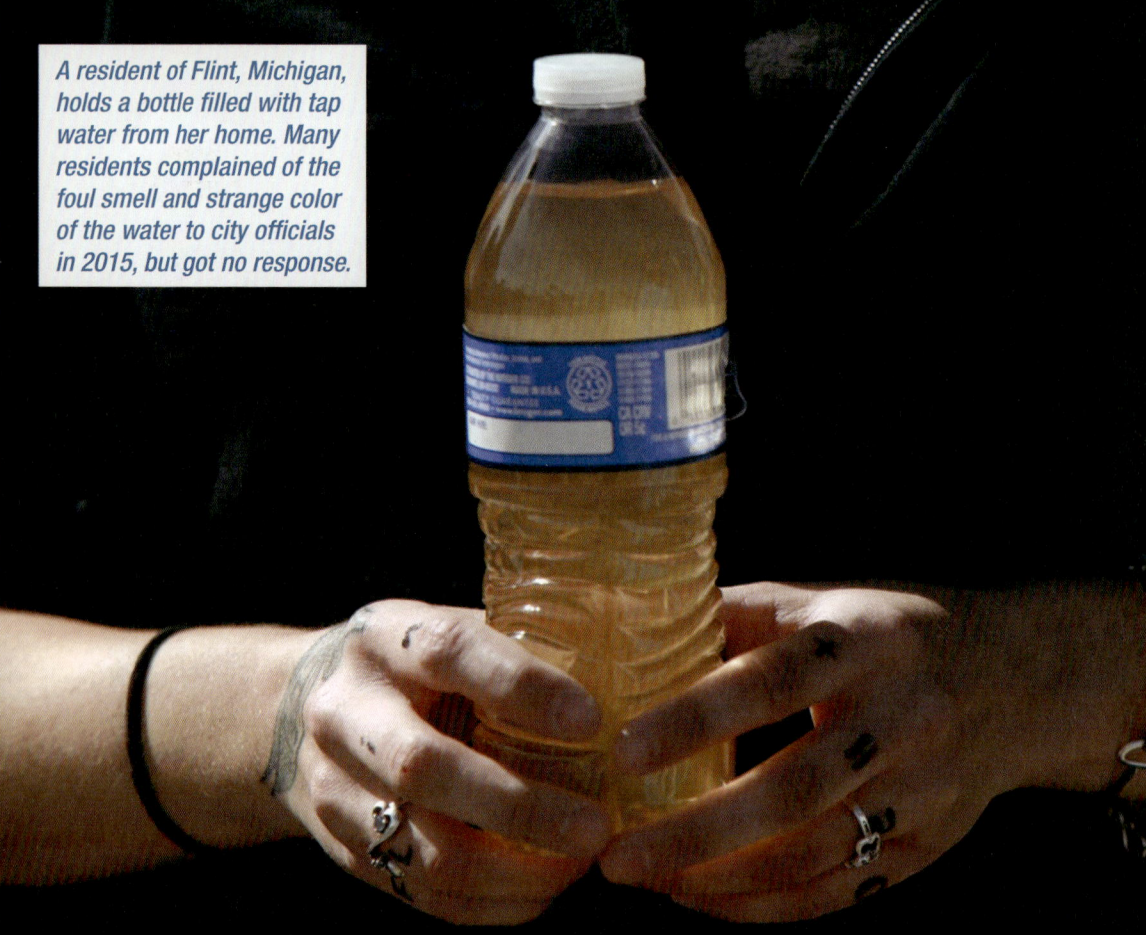

A resident of Flint, Michigan, holds a bottle filled with tap water from her home. Many residents complained of the foul smell and strange color of the water to city officials in 2015, but got no response.

As time went by, it could no longer be denied that lead was an extremely toxic and dangerous substance. During the 1970s US government officials began taking legislative steps to ban most uses of lead, including lead-based paint and leaded gas. But because lead contamination came from so many different sources, it was too late to stop the environmental buildup. As a result, lead contamination remains a serious problem in the United States today—one that experts warn is worse than many people realize.

A Solvable Problem

Largely because of the Flint water crisis and the massive amount of publicity that followed, people are now more aware of the dangers of lead contamination. This became clear during a January–February 2017 poll by the Water Quality Association, which involved more than seventeen hundred adults in the United States. When asked about perceived water contaminants, the number of respondents who cited lead was more than double that in a 2015 poll by the same group. There was also an increase in the number of respondents who said they learned about water contaminants from the media: from 27 percent in 2015 to 43 percent in 2017.

Public health officials now consider lead contamination to be one of the most urgent problems threatening human health, especially children's health. The good news is, the problem can be improved through a combination of increased public awareness, federal and state funding to clean up existing lead contamination, and preventive measures. In the words of New York City physician Elaine Schulte, "Lead poisoning continues to be one of the most preventable public health problems."[4]

> "Lead poisoning continues to be one of the most preventable public health problems."[4]
>
> —Elaine Schulte, a physician from New York City

CHAPTER ONE

Public Health Crises in the Making

The centuries-long mining of lead and its widespread use have taken a heavy toll on the environment and people. Despite drastic reductions in the use of lead, it still contaminates water, air, and soil. Years of research have revealed many different sources of lead contamination, including corroded pipes that allow lead to leach into the water supply, industrial operations, motor vehicles that burn leaded fuel, and lead-based paint, or lead paint, as it is typically known. Of all the sources of lead contamination known to scientists, lead paint is considered one of the most problematic—and most dangerous.

Old Paint, Lingering Dangers

The fact that lead paint is still such a health risk may seem surprising, since it has been banned in the United States since 1978. But legislation only brought an end to new uses of lead paint. By the time it was banned, the paint had been used for nearly a hundred years in homes, apartment buildings, schools, child care centers, and all kinds of other structures throughout the country. Lead paint was widely considered the premier paint for all kinds of uses, as a 1920s ad by the paint company Sherwin-Williams touted: "White lead should be the basic ingredient of all white paint and light tints. It is to these paints exactly what flour is to bread."[5] Walls and doors were coated with lead paint, as were floors, woodwork, stairways, stair railings, and exterior siding and porches.

Even though more than forty years have passed since its ban, a great deal of that lead paint is still around. According to David Jacobs, chief scientist for the National Center for Healthy Housing, some 37 million residences throughout the country contain lead paint. And the older the dwelling, the more such paint that is typically present. Data from the US Environmental Protection Agency (EPA) show that homes built between 1960 and 1977 have a 24 percent chance of containing lead paint. That number jumps to 69 percent for homes built between 1940 and 1959 and to 87 percent for homes built before 1940.

Many people living in older homes believe that if they paint their walls with multiple coats of newer, safer latex paint, the underlying lead paint no longer poses a hazard. And that may be true—as long as the old paint remains completely undisturbed. When people decide to renovate, however, and in the process attempt to get rid of lead paint, they run into problems. "So much lead exposure happens when people do renovations,"[6] says Wendy Heiger-Bernays, associate professor of environmental health at Boston University's School of Public Health.

> "So much lead exposure happens when people do renovations."[6]
>
> —Wendy Heiger-Bernays, associate professor of environmental health at Boston University's School of Public Health

Because of the risk, contractors who work on buildings that have lead paint are required by the EPA to take stringent precautions. Since 2010, with enactment of the Lead Renovation, Repair and Painting Rule (known as the RRP Rule), workers must be certified by the EPA, and property owners and landlords must hire only workers who are certified. This applies to any sort of construction activity that disturbs lead paint, including remodeling, electrical work, window replacement, plumbing, and painting. Those who are caught violating the EPA's rule are subject to thousands of dollars in fines and possible jail time. Yet research has shown that many contractors are either unaware of the RRP Rule or intentionally ignore it. "As a result," says environmental hazards expert Michael Collins, "contractors across the US regularly and needlessly expose the public to unacceptable risks during renovation, repair, and painting efforts."[7]

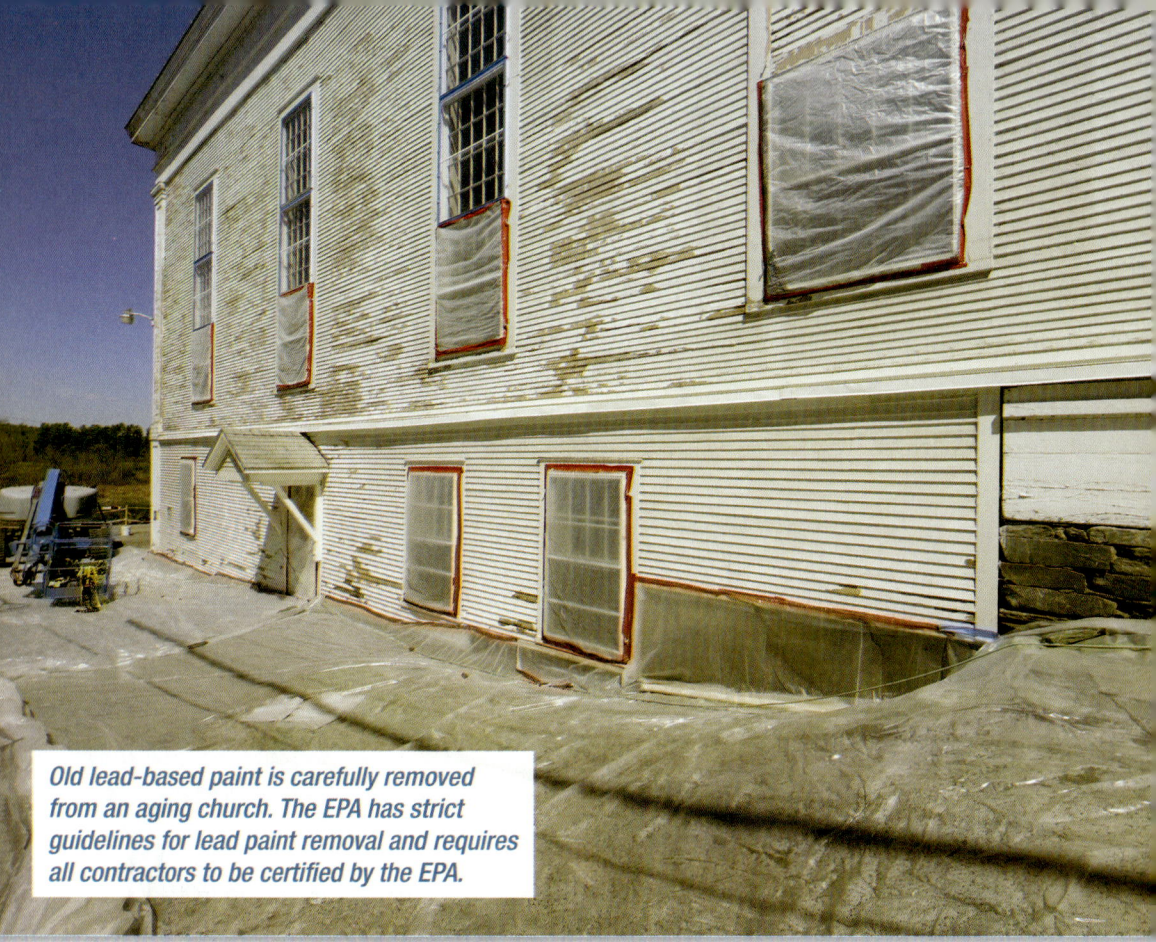

Old lead-based paint is carefully removed from an aging church. The EPA has strict guidelines for lead paint removal and requires all contractors to be certified by the EPA.

Poisonous Dust

A common perception about lead paint is that the biggest risk is for young children to eat paint chips that flake off walls. Although that does happen and is dangerous when it does, it is no longer very common. A far more prevalent source of lead exposure is household dust that has been contaminated by lead paint. In fact, the American Academy of Pediatrics states that lead-contaminated dust is the primary source of lead poisoning among children in the United States.

Lead dust is created when walls and other surfaces coated with lead paint are scraped, sanded—especially with power sanders—or knocked down. Such activities disturb the old paint and send huge amounts of toxic lead dust into the air. The dust accumulates on floors, rugs, countertops, furniture, and other surfaces, and it poses a serious risk for occupants, especially young children. They inhale the toxic dust and also get it on their hands. When they put their hands in their mouths, which all young children do, they are at risk for lead poisoning. Maria Wargovich, a lead specialist from Savannah, Georgia, explains, "At that age, the hand to mouth behavior is a main source of lead poisoning, and it's normal for children to explore their environments by putting things in their mouths."[8]

Sometimes people take every precaution to reduce lead paint dangers in their homes and are shocked to learn the places where deadly lead dust can hide. This was the case with Freddie Mae Slaughter, a resident of Kansas City, Missouri. For nearly twenty years Slaughter has owned an older home in the city. She was aware that there was lead paint on the interior walls, and she coated them several times with bright-white latex paint. Because she cares for a two-year-old child during the week, Slaughter wanted to be sure that her home was safe from lead dangers, so she arranged for contractors to do an inspection. What they found was alarming. As diligent as Slaughter had been about painting over the lead paint on her walls, she had not considered the windowsills between the inside and outside panes, which were also found to be covered in lead paint. The contractors explained that every time she slid her windows up to let fresh air inside and then closed them later, lead dust floated into the house. "People don't know that lead can still be in the windows,"[9] says Slaughter.

> "The hand to mouth behavior is a main source of lead poisoning, and it's normal for children to explore their environments by putting things in their mouths."[8]
>
> —Maria Wargovich, a lead specialist from Savannah, Georgia

Billowing Clouds of Dust

Throughout the United States, lead contamination from renovation and demolition is a serious, persistent problem. This is especially true in older cities with numerous homes and apartment buildings that were constructed years before lead paint was banned. One example is New York City, which is America's most populous city and home to numerous older buildings. Renovation of these buildings is happening constantly, and many of these structures are so old and deteriorated that they require gut renovation. This is a construction term that refers to stripping rooms down to their raw framing and replacing everything from walls and floors to pipes, plumbing, and electrical systems. Old apartment buildings that are gut renovated are invariably filled with surfaces coated in lead paint. If contractors do not use lead-safe construction practices as sanctioned by the EPA—which in many cases they do not—their work generates massive amounts of toxic lead dust. In New York's East Village, for example, some apartments have been found to have lead levels significantly higher than what the federal government considers acceptable.

This was the case at Liz Haak's apartment, where lead levels were found to be at least sixteen times higher than federal limits. At one point, new security cameras were being installed on all floors, which required workers to cut large holes into the walls. Haak saw no plastic tenting or other precautions to contain lead dust, and it filled the air. "It was very careless work, and not supervised by [the landlord]," she says. "When you walked into the building, there's just clouds of dust. . . . I was just furious."[10]

The risk of contamination from lead dust increases dramatically during housing demolitions, such as those taking place in Detroit, Michigan. Detroit is a city that has fought its way back from economic disaster. A severe decline in its population has left more than seventy thousand homes vacant. The homes became havens for squatters, drug dealers, and other criminals, which contributed to widespread deterioration of neighborhoods. To address the problem, Detroit officials applied for federal assistance to demolish the abandoned houses, and in 2014 the request was granted. The city received $50 million to spend on demolition, and as the decrepit houses have disappeared

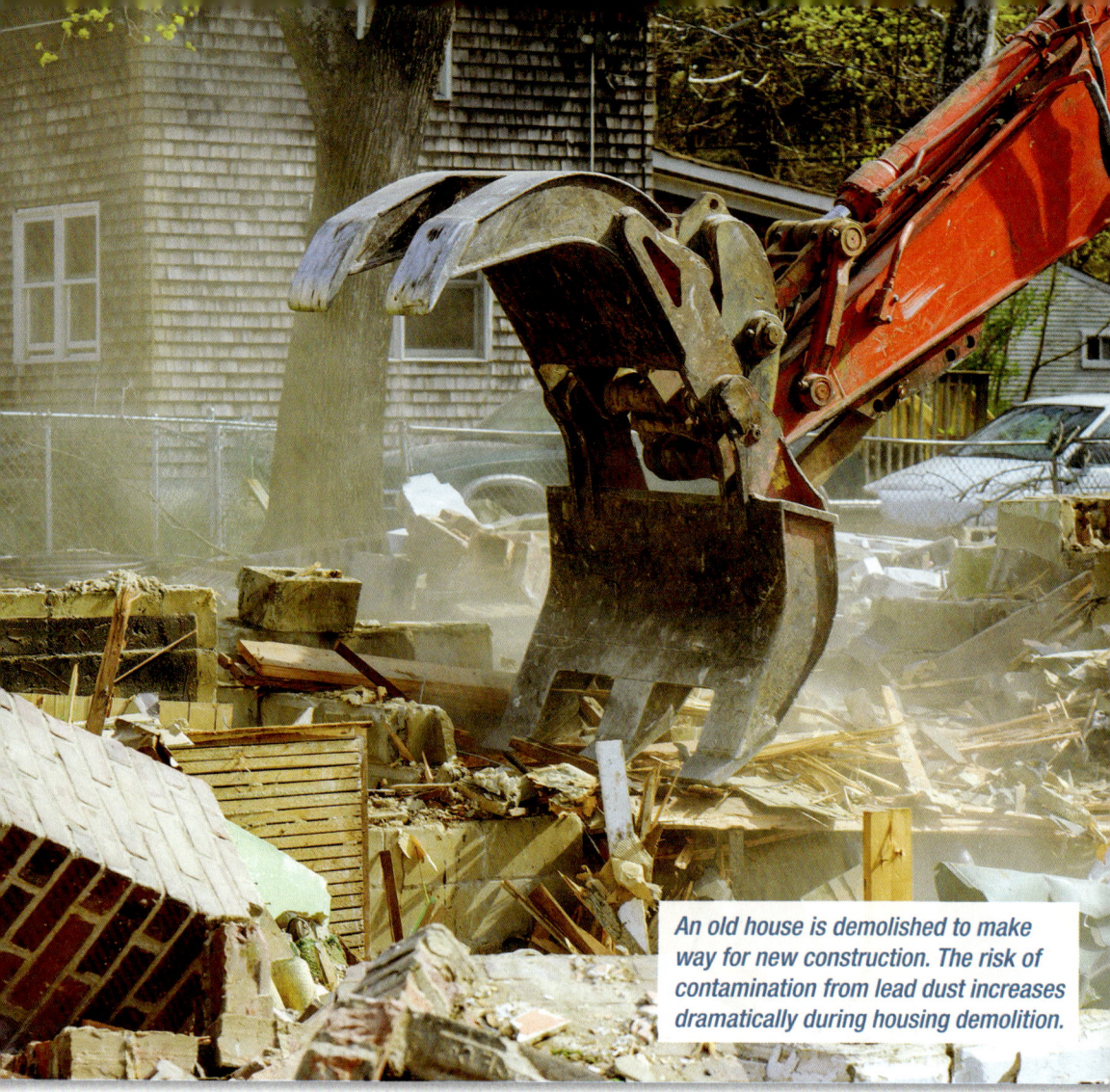

An old house is demolished to make way for new construction. The risk of contamination from lead dust increases dramatically during housing demolition.

one by one, this has improved neighborhoods and eased the minds of residents. But the demolition has also created a new problem: The percentage of children with elevated blood lead levels has increased. Health officials fear that this is because the demolition has spread lead-contaminated dust throughout neighborhoods.

In 2017 the Detroit Health Department conducted a study to examine the blood lead levels of fifty thousand city children. The researchers found that living within 400 feet (122 m) of a demolition site increased the odds of blood lead elevation by 20 percent. Where there were two or more demolitions nearby, the odds increased by 38 percent. "Even one lead poisoned child is one too many," says Detroit Health Department director Joneigh Khaldun. "We have to try something new. If there is a potential association, let's not do [demolitions] at all."[11] On the basis of the discovery, the city halted demolitions in some neighborhoods, pending further study.

How Lead Contaminates Soil

As Detroit's experience demonstrates, large-scale demolitions and renovations of older buildings with lead paint can contaminate the environment. When these buildings are torn down or renovated, enormous clouds of dust fill the air. Eventually the toxic dust settles onto the ground and clings to soil—permanently.

Unlike some substances, lead does not biodegrade (break down) or disappear over time. "Trouble is, lead is forever,"[12] says environmental researcher Michael Ketterer.

> "Trouble is, lead is forever."[12]
>
> —Michael Ketterer, an environmental researcher at Northern Arizona University

One city where widespread housing renovation has contributed to lead-contaminated soil is Oakland, California. According to Larry Brooks, who directs operations for Alameda County's Healthy Homes Department, Oakland has a huge number of older buildings that are coated with crumbling lead paint. This has been a major contributor to the city's problem of soil contamination. "We're finding it often," says Brooks, "as a result of deteriorated paint from the exterior, rain rinses it into the soil and contaminates it."[13]

Soil in Philadelphia, Pennsylvania, has also been contaminated by lead, with large-scale renovation projects cited as a major contributor. This is an especially serious problem in the river wards, which is a cluster of neighborhoods along the banks of the Delaware River. The river wards area has grown more desirable in recent years, which has led to a fivefold increase in construction projects since 2010. During a study in 2017 by two Philadelphia newspapers, investigators tested soil in more than one hundred parks, playgrounds, and backyards in the river wards. Nearly 75 percent of the tested areas were found to have hazardous levels of lead. Investigators also discovered that contractors working on construction projects were not always following lead-safe practices. Although the final report did not blame unsafe construction practices for the lead contamination, it was determined to be a likely contributor. "We found lots of sites with just giant heaping piles of [contaminated] dirt left uncovered, blowing in the wind,"[14] says Wendy Ruderman, a reporter who worked on the investigation.

Lead Found in Baby Food

As publicity related to lead contamination has grown, so has public awareness about the dangers of lead and its sources. Many people now know about children's exposure to lead from contaminated drinking water, as well as the hazards posed by old lead-based paint and soil contaminated by years of vehicles burning leaded gas. What is not so widely known is that food can also be a source of lead—including food made for babies. In June 2017 the Environmental Defense Fund released a report on different types of baby food that were tested as part of a long-term study. Overall, 20 percent of the 2,164 baby food samples were found to contain detectable levels of lead.

The study revealed that fruit juices (grape, mixed fruit, apple, and pear) contained the highest amounts of lead of all baby food. Root vegetables such as sweet potatoes and carrots contained lead, as did arrowroot cookies, teething biscuits, some fruits, prepared meals, and desserts. The researchers say it is not clear whether the lead in baby food came from the soil in which the fruits and vegetables were grown or from another source. And even though none of the lead levels exceeded federal standards, health officials say that no amount of lead is safe for children. "The levels we found were relatively low," says study author Tom Neltner, "but when you add them up—with all the foods children eat—it's significant."

Quoted in Allison Aubrey, "Lead Detected in Baby Food Samples. Pediatricians Say There's No Safe Level," NPR, June 15, 2017. www.npr.org.

Toxic Remnants of the Past

Along with lead-tainted construction dust, experts say other factors are involved in Philadelphia's contaminated soil. One of these is the decades-long burning of leaded gas, which is a known pollutant. The US government began phasing out leaded gasoline during the 1970s and banned it altogether for automobile use in 1996. Still, motor vehicles traveling America's streets, roads, and highways burned it in their engines for more than sixty years. The combustion of leaded gas spewed millions of tons of lead into the atmosphere. Tiny particles of the toxic metal eventually settled onto the ground and contaminated the soil. This contamination was most serious in areas close to roads and highways, as well as in large, heavily trafficked cities like Philadelphia.

Industry is another likely contributor to Philadelphia's soil contamination problem. The city was once home to thirty-six active smelting operations, in which ore was heated to extract the metals inside it. Fourteen of these smelters were located in the river wards. A June 2017 investigative story called "Toxic City" describes the neighborhood when the smelters were active: "It was a time when manufacturers used lead in everything from paints to plastics. Lunch-pail laborers walked to work from tightly packed row homes as lead dust spewed from smokestacks, coating sidewalks, stoops, and yards."[15]

The smelters in Philadelphia closed years ago, but their environmental toxins remained. Researchers say that all neighborhoods near the former lead smelters are likely to have unsafe levels of lead in the soil—and testing has confirmed this. River wards resident Jana Curtis has seen alarming evidence of it herself, since soil samples from her yard were found to be three times higher than the federal maximum. Tests also showed that her little girl had elevated lead levels in her bloodstream. "The yard was poisoning my daughter," says Curtis. "It's just so horrifying."[16]

Water Unfit to Drink

Some of the sources that have contaminated soil with lead have also contaminated water. For instance, precipitation can wash industrial pollutants and remnants of leaded emissions from motor vehicles into lakes and streams and potentially contaminate drinking water. The most common source of lead-contaminated water, however, is leaching from corroded pipes, which is what happened in Flint, Michigan, in 2014.

Flint's water became contaminated after a change in the water supply. City officials had made a budgetary decision to temporarily switch from Flint's longtime supplier (the city of Detroit),

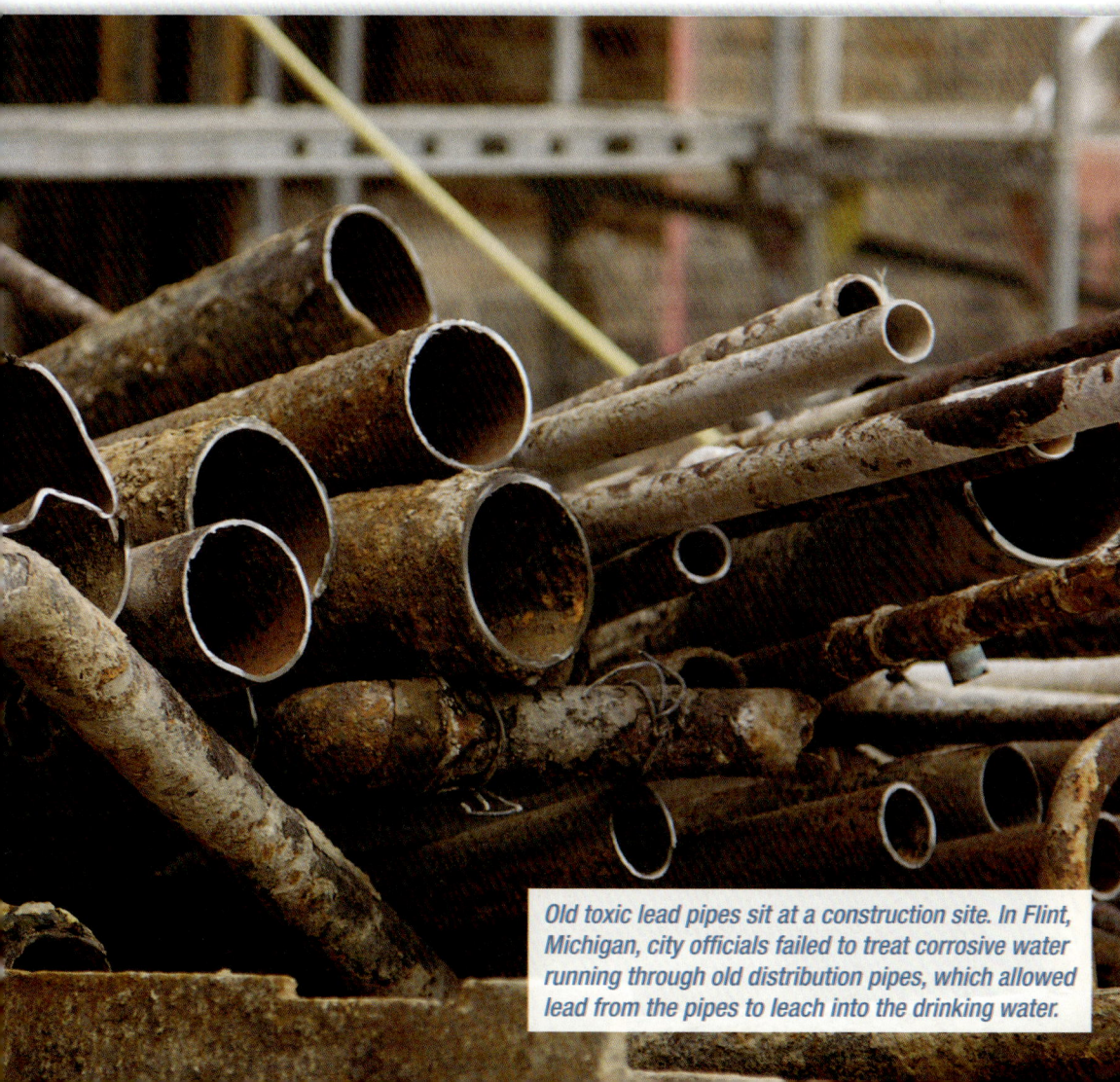

Old toxic lead pipes sit at a construction site. In Flint, Michigan, city officials failed to treat corrosive water running through old distribution pipes, which allowed lead from the pipes to leach into the drinking water.

which furnished pretreated water from Lake Huron, to the Flint River. The river water was polluted and known to be highly corrosive, but this was treatable with an anticorrosion substance known as orthophosphate. Flint officials, however, intentionally opted to skip the treatment in order to cut costs. As a result, the corrosive water began eating away at the insides of aging water distribution pipes, which allowed lead from the pipes to leach into the water. Although Flint officials denied for more than a year that the water was contaminated, they finally had to face what they had done. Their decision proved to be catastrophic and was also deemed criminal. Thousands of Flint's children were exposed to

Toxic Toys

When parents give their children toys to play with, it is natural for them to assume that the toys are safe. If they are made in the United States and are relatively new, then they are likely safe. In 1978 the US government banned the use of lead in house paint, as well as in any products marketed for children, including toys. But older toys may still represent a potential hazard for children, as the EPA explains: "That favorite dump truck or rocking chair handed down in the family, antique doll furniture, or toy jewelry could contain lead-based paint or contain lead in the material it is made from." Children can also be exposed to lead through toys that are imported from China—which accounts for an estimated 80 percent of all toys sold in the United States.

The Consumer Product Safety Commission (CPSC) is the federal agency charged with monitoring imported toys and issuing recalls if the lead content in toys exceeds more than the trace amount allowed by US law. In August 2018 the CPSC issued a recall alert for tens of thousands of Rubber Critters, which are often used to play toss and catch games. The toys are imported from China and come in various colors and animal shapes, including alligators, chickens, frogs, fish, pigs, penguins, cows, and octopuses. CPSC inspections found that orange and yellow surface paint used on the toys contains lead levels that violate US regulations.

US Environmental Protection Agency, "Protect Your Family from Exposures to Lead," August 30, 2017. www.epa.gov.

lead-contaminated water, and it may be many years before the extent of their health damage is known.

In October 2018 news reports revealed water contamination in Newark, New Jersey. As in Flint, Newark officials continuously insisted that there was no problem and the water was fine. "The parallels to Flint are fairly clear," says Erik Olson, an official with the Natural Resources Defense Council. "The city was denying a problem even though its own data was showing problems."[17] Although Newark's water contamination problem was not as extreme as Flint's, it was still found to be significant.

Newark officials were first alerted about lead contamination of the water in 2017, when the state began testing water systems in a number of New Jersey cities, including Newark. More than 22 percent of the samples tested higher than the federal government's maximum for lead content in water. City officials downplayed the risk and assured residents that there was nothing to worry about. "NEWARK'S WATER IS ABSOLUTELY SAFE TO DRINK,"[18] the city's website declared. Then, during the summer of 2018, the Natural Resources Defense Council filed a lawsuit against the city. The lawsuit alleged that city officials had failed to properly treat water with anticorrosive chemicals, which had allowed lead to leach into the water supply.

Newark officials abruptly changed course and announced a giveaway of forty thousand water filters to residents. Officials also stated that the method for treating water would be changed to remedy the lead contamination problem. In an October 2018 news conference, Newark mayor Ras Baraka stated, "If we don't have corrosion control measures that effectively reduce the amount of lead that's going into people's water before we change their lead service lines, we need to act."[19]

A Public Health Issue of Urgency

Lead contamination is a complex, threatening problem with numerous causes. Decades ago US government officials acknowledged that lead paint was dangerous, and it was banned. Later

> "It remains a public health priority to continue reducing lead exposure, especially in highly-exposed communities."[20]
>
> —The EPA, an agency of the US government whose mission is to protect human and environmental health

the same acknowledgment was made about leaded gas and its pollution of the environment, and it was also banned. Industries whose emissions and waste were found to be toxic to the environment were shut down. These and other such actions have made a dramatic difference, since lead in the air and water has significantly declined. Blood tests among children have shown that on average, lead levels have also declined over the years. Yet even with the progress that has been made, lead contamination is not a thing of the past. This toxic metal still contaminates the air, water, soil, and dust, and in the process, it puts human lives at risk—with young children having the greatest risk of all. "It remains a public health priority," says the EPA, "to continue reducing lead exposure, especially in highly-exposed communities."[20]

CHAPTER TWO

A Heavy Toll on Human Health

It is a fact that certain types of metal are essential for human health. Iron, for instance, is necessary for the body to produce a protein that creates red blood cells, which then carry oxygen from the lungs throughout the body. Chromium helps maintain normal blood sugar levels, and zinc helps blood clot and bolsters the immune system. Copper, magnesium, calcium, and several other metals also play important roles in keeping people healthy—but the same is not true of lead. "Lead is a true poison that has no necessary role in the body,"[21] says Mary Gearing, a molecular biologist from Boston, Massachusetts. In fact, research has clearly shown that exposure to even small amounts of lead can cause severe health problems and damage that lasts a lifetime.

> "Lead is a true poison that has no necessary role in the body."[21]
>
> —Mary Gearing, a molecular biologist from Boston, Massachusetts

How Lead Affects the Body

Lead is known for being extremely harmful to humans, but exactly how it affects the body is not common knowledge. "News reports rarely discuss the biology behind lead poisoning,"[22] says Gearing. She goes on to explain that lead's dangerous potential stems from its ability to mimic and disrupt essential molecules in the body. It interferes with the normal functions of cells, which are the basic building blocks of all living things. When lead gets into the body, it begins to displace beneficial metals such as calcium, zinc, and iron. In particular, lead targets calcium because the two are chemically similar. Lead disrupts the movement and storage of calcium inside cells, which increases cell stress and can lead to the death of brain cells known as neurons. Gearing explains, "Because it looks . . . a lot like calcium, an essential player in brain chemistry, lead can sneak into the otherwise well-protected brain."[23]

By "well-protected brain," Gearing is referring to a protective network of blood vessels and tissue known as the blood-brain barrier. This barrier's function is to keep toxins and infectious substances that may be circulating in the blood from getting into the brain and causing harm to the central nervous system. The blood-brain barrier is highly effective at protecting the brain but is semipermeable, which means some substances can cross through but others cannot. Lead, unfortunately, is one substance that can penetrate the blood-brain barrier. Scientists attribute this to lead's chemical similarity to (and ability to mimic) calcium.

Children Most Vulnerable

People of all ages can be harmed by lead exposure. Adults can develop a number of health problems, including digestive disorders, muscle and joint pain, dizziness, and headaches. By far, however, lead contamination poses the greatest risk to children, especially children who are younger than six. That is why, says Flint physician Mona Hanna-Attisha, "When pediatricians hear anything about lead, we absolutely freak out."[24]

> "When pediatricians hear anything about lead, we absolutely freak out."[24]
>
> —Mona Hanna-Attisha, the physician from Flint, Michigan, who sounded the alarm on the city's water crisis

Children are especially vulnerable to the effects of lead because their bodies and brains are still developing. The first six years (and especially the first three years) of life is when a child's brain grows the fastest. It is during this time that the brain forms critical connections that control thinking, learning, memory, movement, behavior, and emotions. According to physician Bruce P. Lanphear, an internationally recognized expert on lead and other

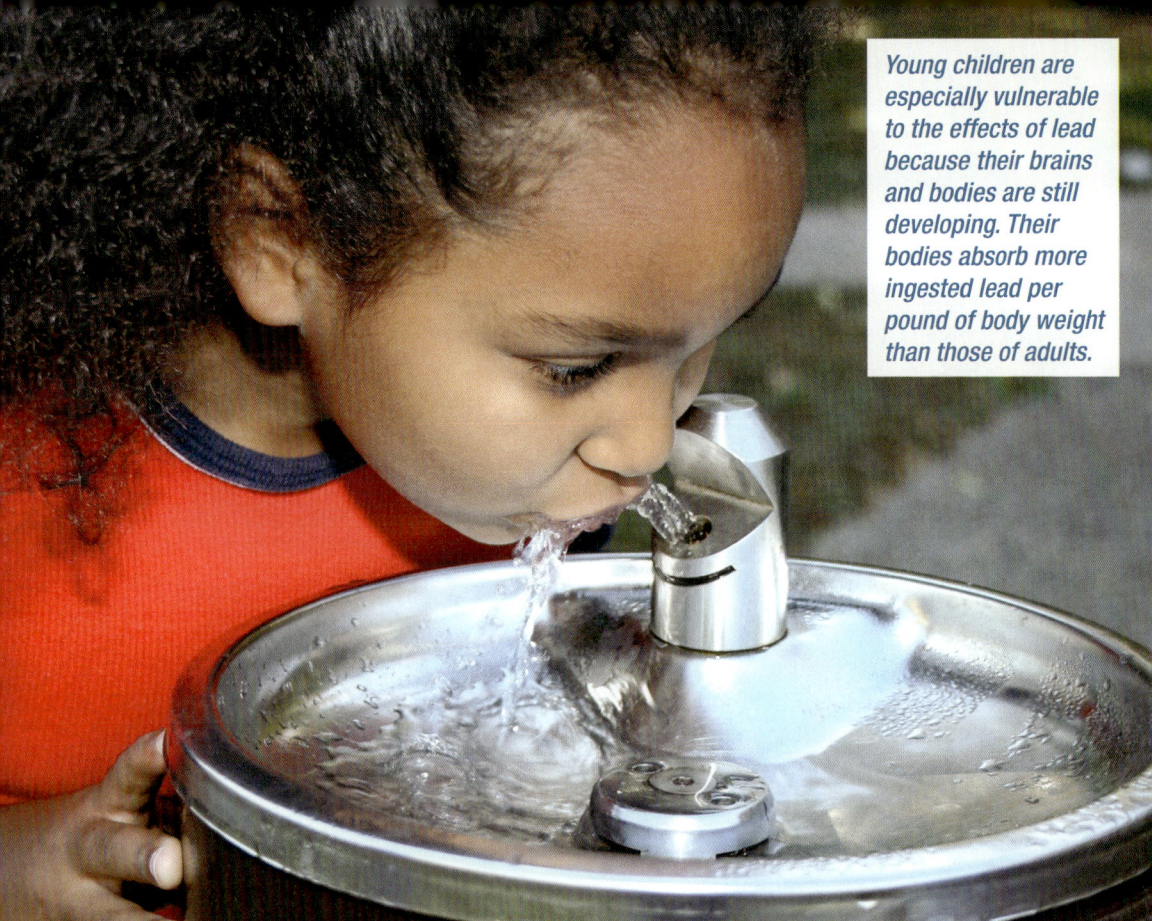

Young children are especially vulnerable to the effects of lead because their brains and bodies are still developing. Their bodies absorb more ingested lead per pound of body weight than those of adults.

neurotoxins, growing cells in a child's nervous system are more vulnerable to toxins than fully formed cells. Thus, says Lanphear, "the brain is particularly vulnerable to lead exposure during early childhood."[25]

Another reason for young children's vulnerability to lead is related to the size of their bodies. Because they are small and their bodies are growing, they absorb more ingested lead per pound than adults who are exposed to the same environmental toxins. When children under age six ingest lead, for instance, an estimated 50 percent is absorbed by their bodies. Comparatively, 5 percent to 10 percent of lead is absorbed by older children, and even less than that is absorbed by adults. "The absorption of lead is much, much higher in young children," says pediatrician Kanta J. Bhambhani, who directs the Lead Poisoning Clinic at Children's Hospital of Michigan. "And of course the effects are also greater

> ### Lead Exposure Affects Fertility
>
> Scientists have long known about a connection between lead exposure and infertility. Old medical journals chronicle the use of lead pills by women who wanted to terminate pregnancies. Also, women who worked with lead in factory jobs were found to be less likely to conceive than women without such exposure. Current research, such as a 2018 study, has confirmed the link between lead exposure and fertility. The study involved examining data on airborne lead from 1978 to 1988 (when leaded gas was being phased out), and data on topsoil during the early 2000s. The researchers also examined birth statistics for both periods of time.
>
> One discovery was that as atmospheric lead levels declined over the decade from 1978 to 1988, fertility rates increased by 4.5 births per 1,000 women. But during the early 2000s, areas with high lead concentrations in topsoil experienced a significant drop in fertility rates: a decrease of 7.8 births per 1,000 women. The topsoil finding was the most troubling to the researchers because, as they explain in the May 2018 report, "it suggests that lead may continue to impair fertility today, both in the United States and in other countries that have significant amounts of lead in topsoil."
>
> Karen Clay et al., "Toxic Truth: Lead and Fertility," IZA Discussion Paper No. 11541, May 30, 2018. https://papers.ssrn.com.

in younger children. The risk is greatest at less than 6 years of age, and the younger the child, the greater the risk."[26]

One of the most obvious and understandable reasons for children's vulnerability to lead is that they have more direct exposure to it than adults. The younger children are, the more time they spend crawling around on floors and exploring their world by putting objects they find in their mouths. If there are chips of lead paint or lead-contaminated dust in their environment, the risk for lead ingestion is especially high for these youngsters.

Because children are so vulnerable to harm from lead exposure, the Centers for Disease Control and Prevention (CDC) has lowered its reference level (sometimes called level of concern) for lead content in children's blood. The purpose of the CDC's reference level is to identify children whose blood lead levels are much higher than most children's levels. Blood tests for lead are measured in micrograms (one-millionth of a gram) of lead per deciliter (one-tenth of a liter) of blood. Before 2012 the CDC's reference level was 10 micrograms per deciliter (mcg/dL), and since 2012 it has been 5 mcg/dL. This measurement does not indicate a level that is acceptable or safe, since there is no such thing. "The only safe lead level is no lead,"[27] says Howard Markel, a physician with the University of Michigan School of Public Health.

A Tiny Victim of Lead Poisoning

Since it is widely known that even a small amount of lead is harmful for children, the extraordinarily high blood lead level of a little Washington, DC, girl was both shocking and alarming to health officials. When two-year-old Heavenz Luster was tested for lead in 2016, her blood lead level was 120 mcg/dL—twenty-four times higher than what the CDC considers elevated. It was the worst case of lead poisoning city health officials had seen in more than twenty years.

In July 2016 Heavenz and her family moved into a home in Washington, DC. Because the home had been built in 1923, its walls were covered in lead paint. City records showed that the home had a history of peeling paint, and the owner had been cited for not taking care of the issue. He insisted that he had finally made the necessary repairs, an inspector approved the home for rental, and the Lusters moved in. They had been homeless, so having their own place seemed like a dream come true—until three months later.

Heavenz's parents had been watching her closely and knew that something was terribly wrong. The little girl stopped interacting with her family and seemed to close herself into a world only she could see. When someone spoke her name, she did not respond. She spoke no words, screamed loudly for no apparent reason, seemed anxious much of the time, and rocked from side to side. Her parents took her to a doctor, and blood tests confirmed that Heavenz suffered from severe lead poisoning. She immediately underwent treatment to clear the lead from her system, but any damage that was done to her brain is likely permanent. "Once you're lead poisoned, you're lead poisoned for life," says Daniel Levy, a pediatrician who has treated numerous children for lead poisoning. In reference to Heavenz, he says, "It's not a death sentence, necessarily, but it doesn't bode well for [her] future."[28]

Although no one knows exactly what the future holds for Heavenz, scientists have observed how dramatically children's lives can be affected by lead exposure. Lead has been linked to a host of serious health issues among children. These include problems with cognitive skills, memory, and learning, as well as the development of attention-deficit/hyperactivity disorder (ADHD). Dyslexia and other learning disabilities have been observed in children with high blood lead levels, as have shortened attention span and behavioral problems. The younger children are when their bodies and brains are exposed to lead, the greater the risk for these sorts of life-altering problems.

Dangers During Pregnancy

In fact, children can be harmed by lead even before they are born. This occurs when a pregnant woman is exposed to high levels of lead, such as by drinking lead-contaminated water or inhaling lead-contaminated dust in an older home or apartment. Although the placenta's function during pregnancy is to filter out infectious agents and toxic substances that could harm the fetus, it cannot filter out metals such as lead. As a result, lead absorbed by the mother crosses through a layer of protective tissue known as the placental barrier and can enter the body and brain of the developing fetus. The risks when this happens are immense: brain damage to the fetus, premature birth, and even fetal death, which is also called miscarriage.

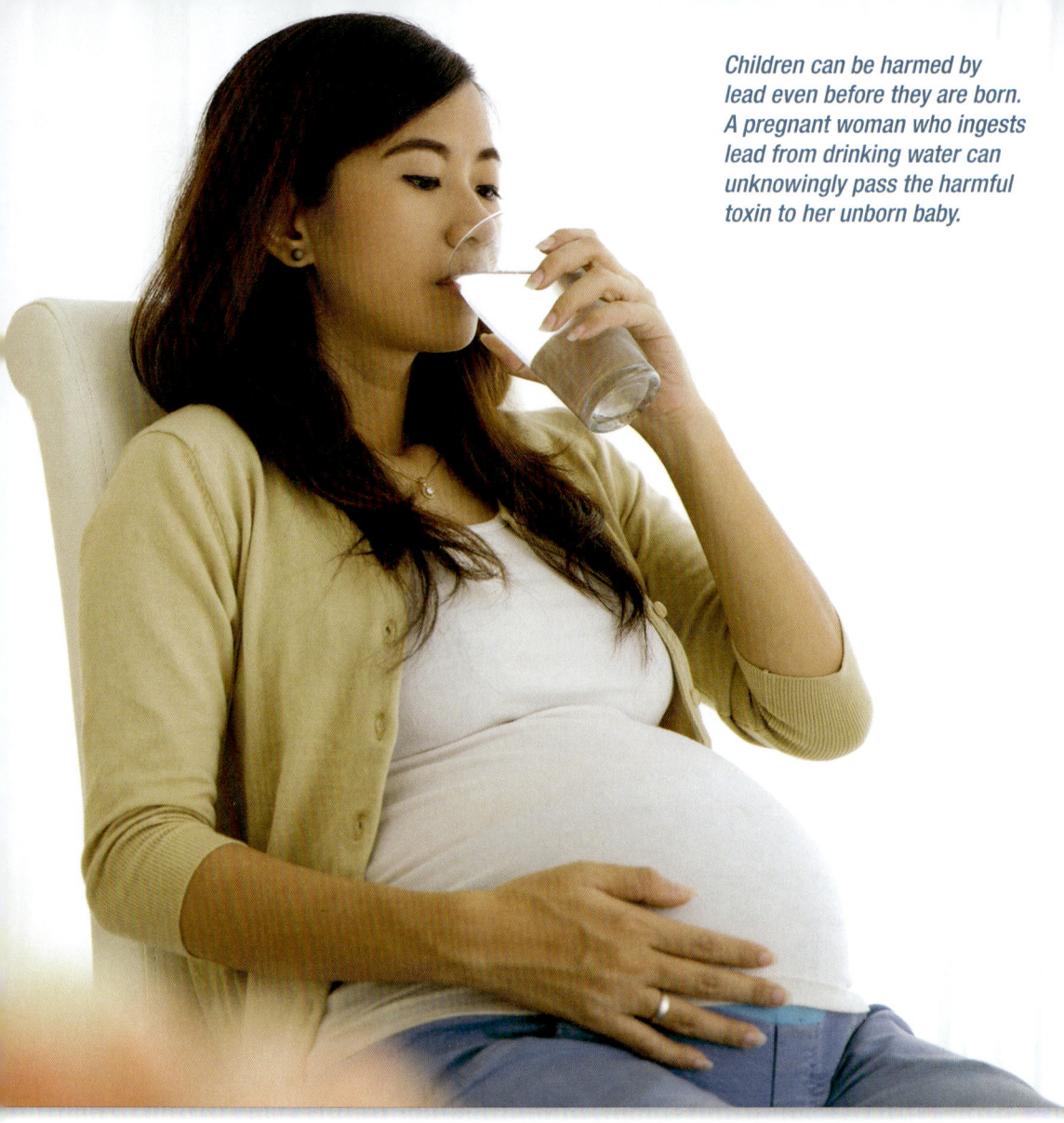

Children can be harmed by lead even before they are born. A pregnant woman who ingests lead from drinking water can unknowingly pass the harmful toxin to her unborn baby.

    An August 2017 study found that the rate of miscarriage rose by 58 percent among pregnant women in Flint who were exposed to lead in the drinking water. The study was conducted by researchers David Slusky of the University of Kansas and Daniel Grossman of West Virginia University. They analyzed women's health records, birth certificates, and fetal death statistics for two time periods: before Flint's source of water changed and after the change, when residents drank the lead-contaminated water. They could clearly see a dramatic 58 percent spike in

> ### Scary News About Adult Lead Exposure
>
> Children are far more vulnerable to being harmed by lead than are adults. But the toxic metal poses risks for people of all ages, and a 2018 study revealed that the risk to adults is greater than researchers had earlier believed. Led by Bruce P. Lanphear, a physician and internationally recognized expert on lead, the researchers set out to determine how much of a role lead exposure played in the deaths of people who died prematurely from cardiovascular disease, coronary artery disease, and other causes. They concluded that nearly 412,000 deaths each year in the United States can be attributed to lead contamination—which is ten times higher than what had been previously estimated.
>
> Nearly 14,300 adults participated in the study, and 90 percent had previously been exposed to lead. The participants were tracked over a period of nearly twenty years. By the end of the study, 4,422 of them had died. On the basis of the cause of death, the researchers concluded that people with the highest blood lead levels had a 37 percent greater risk of dying prematurely from any cause, 70 percent greater risk of dying prematurely from cardiovascular disease, and double the risk of dying from coronary artery disease, compared with people with low blood lead blood levels. "In our study," the authors write, "the estimated number of deaths from all causes and cardiovascular disease that were attributable to concentrations of lead in blood were surprisingly large; indeed, they were comparable with the number of deaths from current tobacco smoke exposure."
>
> Bruce P. Lanphear et al., "Low-Level Lead Exposure and Mortality in US Adults: A Population-Based Cohort Study," *Lancet Public Health*, March 2018. www.thelancet.com.

miscarriage. Slusky and Grossman refer to the Flint fetal death rate as "horrifyingly large" and state that their study provides "robust evidence of the effect of lead on the health of not just infants, but on the health of potential newborns in utero."[29]

Research has also revealed that children born to women who were exposed to lead during pregnancy may develop permanent physical problems such as stunted growth. To examine this, a team of American researchers studied a large group of pregnant women in Mexico City from July 2007 to February 2011. Mexico was chosen because lead exposure is much more common there than in the United States. The primary source of lead exposure for Mexican people is the ceramic dishes and cookware they use for food preparation, serving, and storage. These items are coated with a glaze that has a very high lead content. Along with this pottery, other sources of lead for people in Mexico include cosmetics, the workplace, air pollutants, and drinking water.

The researchers collected blood lead levels from the participants during their second and third trimesters of pregnancy. Blood samples were also taken when the babies were delivered, when they were one month old, and again about four years later. In addition, the researchers measured the children's height, weight, body mass index, and body fat percentage when the children were aged four to six years. The study revealed that the women's high lead exposure during pregnancy was significantly associated with decreased height and weight among their children. In their January 2017 published report, the study authors write, "Lead exposure during pregnancy remains a public health problem with potential lifelong impacts on children's growth and development."[30]

The Tragic Effect of Lead Exposure on Intelligence

When physicians and health officials express concern about lead exposure during pregnancy or early childhood, they invariably focus on the possibility of long-term brain damage and what that could mean for a child's future. Especially troubling is that lead exposure among children has been shown to lower their IQ, which stands for intelligence quotient. In general, the higher the IQ score, the greater someone's intelligence and ability to reason. A large body of scientific research has shown that even low-level lead exposure can rob children of IQ points, and high exposure can have devastating effects.

On average, says Lanphear, a child with blood lead levels greater than 5 mcg/dL loses about six IQ points. Children with blood lead levels between 2.1 and 5 mcg/dL will lose about one and one-half points. Hanna-Attisha says that when she thinks about the children of Flint having to deal with lower IQs because of the contaminated water they drank, it makes it hard to sleep at night. "Imagine what we've done to an entire population," she says. "We've shifted that IQ curve down. We've lost our high achievers, the next kid who's going to be a neurosurgeon, and we have all these children who may now need remedial services."[31]

A report that came out in 2018 appeared to confirm Hanna-Attisha's worst fears about Flint's children. A state government review of schoolchildren's reading proficiency found that reading

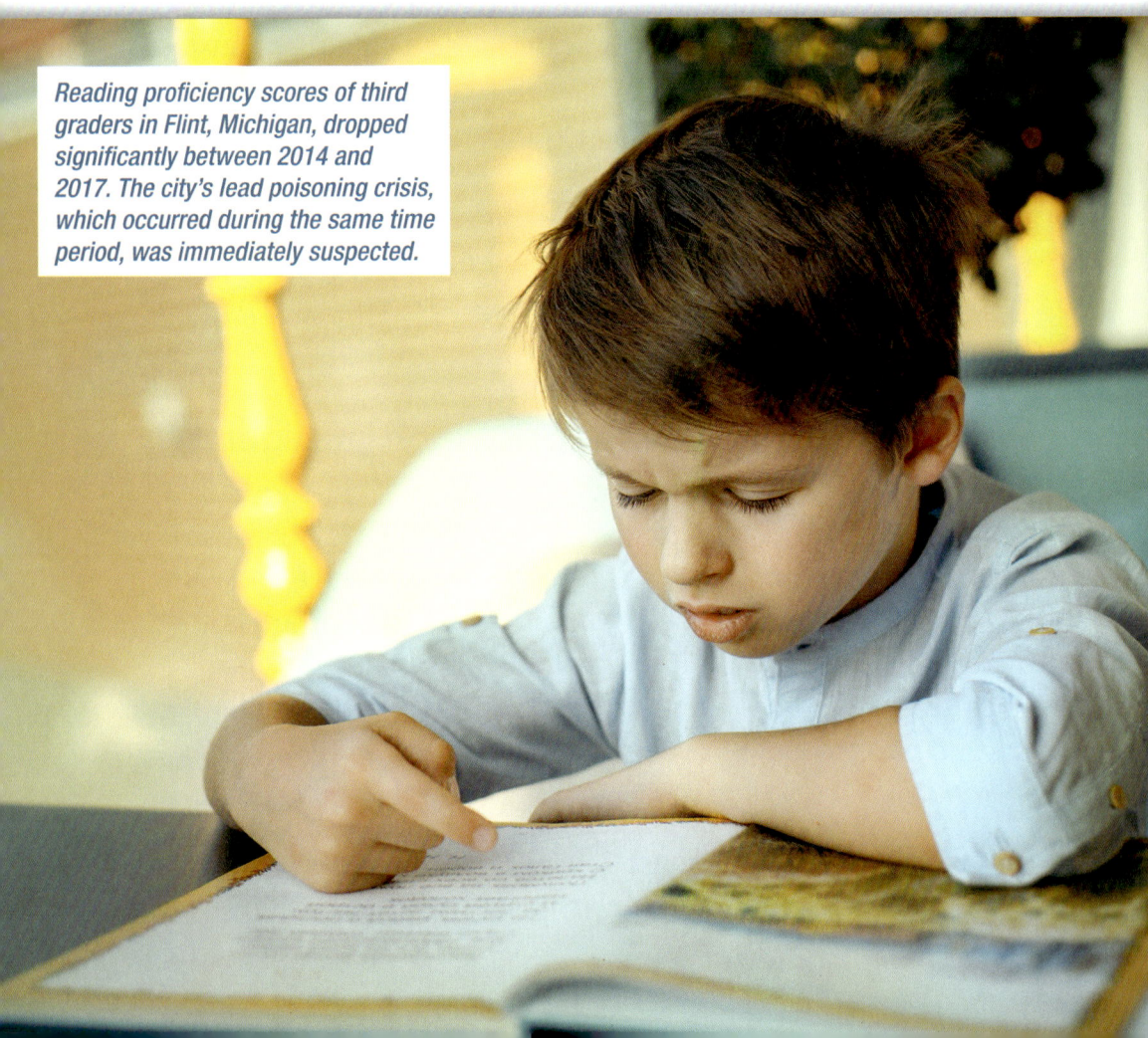

Reading proficiency scores of third graders in Flint, Michigan, dropped significantly between 2014 and 2017. The city's lead poisoning crisis, which occurred during the same time period, was immediately suspected.

levels among the city's third graders had plummeted. In 2014, for instance, nearly 42 percent of third graders had satisfactory reading levels, and by 2017 the number had dropped to just 10.7 percent. Because the lead contamination water crisis happened during that same time period, when the third graders were four or five years old, lead poisoning was immediately suspected. Yet a number of factors could have played a role in the declining reading level, so no one could say with absolute certainty that the children's lead exposure caused the problem. Pediatrician Philip Landrigan, a global expert on lead and one of the first scientists to show how the toxic metal causes brain damage in children, explains, "We know there's a million things that can interfere with reading scores in school—everything from the quality of schools to the quality of homes kids come from. Even though I'm a firm believer that lead is terrible for kids, I don't feel comfortable saying lead caused it." Still, Landrigan adds, "I can tell you with absolute assurance that lead damages children's brains."[32]

> "I can tell you with absolute assurance that lead damages children's brains."[32]
>
> —Philip Landrigan, a pediatrician and global expert on lead

Developmental Disabilities

The harm that lead can cause to a young child's developing brain has also been linked to developmental disabilities. These are conditions that involve impairment in areas of physical development, learning, language, or behavior. If children are not meeting the developmental milestones for their age (such as crawling, walking, and talking) or seem to be regressing, they might have a developmental disability. These disabilities typically begin to develop before birth, such as when a pregnant woman is exposed to lead and it passes through the placenta to the fetus. In other cases, such as when a child is exposed to infectious agents or toxins, the disabilities can develop after a child is born.

A child named John Cale "JC" Brown Jr. began showing signs of a developmental disorder when he was a toddler. JC lived with his parents on an army base in Fort Benning, Georgia. His father, John Cale Brown Sr., was a US Army colonel and battalion commander. When he was promoted in rank, his position required him to live on base in one of the homes that were rented to military families. In 2011 the Brown family moved into a stately white stucco residence that had been home to generations of army families—one that, as it turns out, was seriously contaminated with lead paint.

Before the Browns moved in, JC's mother, Darlena, had inquired about lead paint because the home was eighty years old. She was assured by the rental agent that there was no problem and she had nothing to worry about. The Browns had no reason to doubt the agent's truthfulness until JC began to show disturbing symptoms. At ten months old he had been a happy and outgoing baby, babbling a dozen words and starting to eat different types of foods. By eighteen months he had changed into a different child. He woke up screaming in the night, refused to eat, stopped responding to his name, and no longer used the words he had learned. "He was disappearing into an isolated brain,"[33] says Darlena.

Doctors were mystified by JC's symptoms, wondering if he suffered from severe colic, chronic ear infections, or maybe autism. Finally, in late 2012 when JC was two years old, his pediatrician informed the Browns that the toddler had high levels of lead in his blood. His medical records stated that lead had damaged JC's brain and caused a developmental disorder. An inspection of the home where the Browns had been living found at least 113 spots with cracking, peeling, or crumbling lead paint—and JC's bedroom was one of the problem spots.

As of August 2018, JC was eight years old and had made progress through years of therapy. He continued to struggle with speech, social interactions, and hyperactivity, but he excelled at reading and swimming. He will undoubtedly keep making progress as time goes by, but developmental disorders are not temporary conditions, and he will likely have struggles throughout his life. "I'm sad that my son lost his future," says Darlena. "It was because of where we were that this happened."[34]

An Issue of Vital Concern

What happened to JC Brown is a stark and tragic reminder of the dangers posed by lead, especially the harm it can cause to the brains and bodies of babies and young children. Lead exposure has been linked to a frightening array of health issues, from cognitive problems, impaired memory, stunted growth, and decreased IQ to learning disabilities, behavioral disorders, ADHD, and developmental disabilities—the list goes on and on. Decades of research have broadened scientific knowledge about lead and the many problems it can cause, and this has reinforced health officials' fears about the metal's threats to the public. Jay Schneider, a neuroscientist from Philadelphia, expresses this: "As we learn more about lead and its effects on the brain . . . [we find that] if anything it's even more dangerous than we thought."[35]

> "As we learn more about lead and its effects on the brain . . . [we find that] if anything it's even more dangerous than we thought."[35]
>
> —Jay Schneider, a neuroscientist from Philadelphia

CHAPTER THREE

No End in Sight

Since the 1970s the United States has made noteworthy progress in addressing its lead contamination problem. Legislative efforts to ban leaded gasoline and lead paint, outlaw the use of lead pipes and plumbing fixtures, and slash industrial lead emissions have significantly reduced lead in the air and water. As a result, childhood blood lead levels have steadily declined over the years. Federal health statistics show that the median concentration of lead in the blood of American children aged one to five dropped from 15 mcg/dL in the late 1970s to 0.7 mcg/dL in 2014—a decrease of 95 percent. "The dramatic reduction of blood lead levels in children over the last few decades is a public health triumph,"[36] says Virginia Tech environmental engineer and lead expert Marc Edwards. He emphasizes, however, that the problem is far from resolved.

Despite the reduction in blood levels overall, an alarmingly high number of children still have elevated levels of lead in their blood. According to the CDC, more than five hundred thousand American children aged one to five have blood lead levels greater than 5 mcg/dL. That does not include babies aged one to twelve months, nor does it include older children, so the number is undoubtedly much higher than the CDC estimates. "Childhood lead poisoning has still not been eliminated and further work is clearly needed,"[37] says Edwards. From millions of homes and apartments with lead-based paint on the walls to lead in drinking water to lead-contaminated soil in children's play areas, lead contamination remains a serious problem throughout the United States—one for which there appears to be no end in sight.

Filling a Critical Information Gap

Adding to the problem of lead contamination in the United States is the fact that comprehensive statistics on lead exposure do not exist. There has been no nationwide effort to gather information, largely because such an undertaking would be exorbitantly expensive. The federal government has not allocated funding for such a massive project, nor have government officials even acknowledged that it is needed.

To accumulate data on American children's blood lead levels, the CDC relies on state health departments to report current information. But only ten states and the District of Columbia require universal blood screening for lead among young children, so the CDC's information is spotty at best. All children enrolled in Medicaid are required to receive blood lead screenings at one year and again at two years of age, but this is often not enforced. "Data tracking testing rates and results from the CDC, Medicaid and many state health agencies is incomplete and unreliable," Reuters investigative reporters Joshua Schneyer and M.B. Pell write. "The CDC said its own tracking of lead poisoning rates isn't conclusive, citing insufficient data from states and changes in testing patterns that make comparisons over time challenging."[38]

In an effort to fill this information gap, in 2016 the news organization Reuters embarked on its own investigation. A team of reporters, including Schneyer and Pell, studied lead-related data on communities throughout the United States that was gathered from the CDC and state health departments (not all were willing to cooperate). Then the reporters identified and mapped more than thirty-eight hundred communities where children have abnormally high blood lead levels. Their research revealed that in eleven hundred of those communities, children's blood lead levels were four times

> "Childhood lead poisoning has still not been eliminated and further work is clearly needed."[37]
>
> —Marc Edwards, an environmental engineer and lead expert from Virginia Tech University

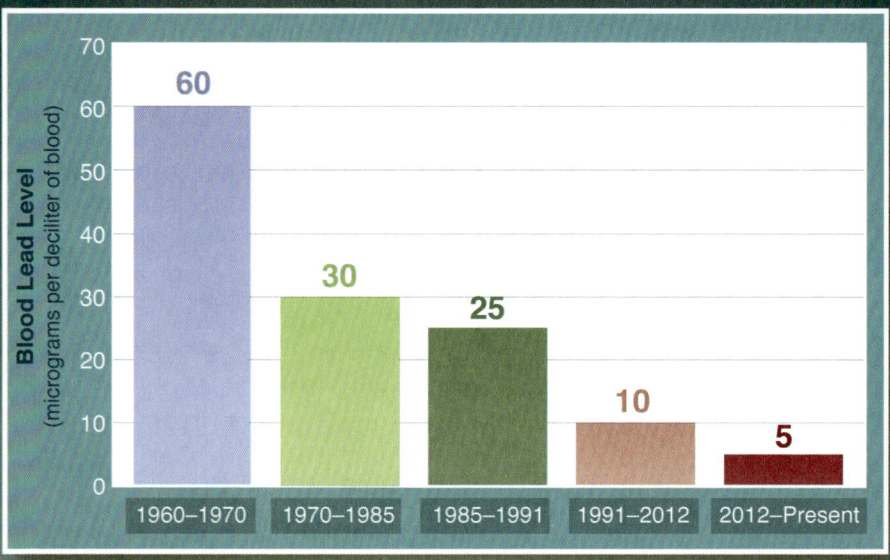

higher than those found in Flint at the height of the water crisis. In the December 2016 report of their findings, Schneyer and Pell write:

> The poisoned places on this map stretch from Warren, Pennsylvania, a town on the Allegheny River where 36 percent of children tested had high lead levels, to a zip code on Goat Island, Texas, where a quarter of tests showed poisoning. In some pockets of Baltimore, Cleveland and Philadelphia, where lead poisoning has spanned generations, the rate of elevated tests over the last decade was 40–50 percent.[39]

Philadelphia was one major Pennsylvania city where children's blood lead levels were abnormally high. The investigation found that in forty-nine different areas known as census tracts, ranging from inner-city Philadelphia to the capital city of Harrisburg, at least 40 percent of children tested for lead had high levels in their blood. In fact, of all the US states, Pennsylvania had the most census tracts—more than eleven hundred—where at least 10 percent of children had elevated blood lead levels. This was alarming to health officials but not surprising. "I believe that," says Loren Robinson, Pennsylvania's deputy secretary for health promotion and disease prevention. "Beyond the history of industry, our state has some of the oldest homes in the country."[40]

Distressing Revelations

Among the worst problem areas identified in the Reuters investigation was St. Joseph, Missouri, a city that is filled with century-old homes with old lead paint on the interior and exterior. From 2010 to 2015, more than 15 percent of children in St. Joseph had elevated blood lead levels, which was triple the state's average of 5 percent. In talking with residents, the investigators learned that many were not aware of the dangers of renovating older homes with lead paint, and some denied that there was a risk at all. According to certified lead inspector Gerald McCush, someone from his office tried to explain to one family that sanding paint off their older home's walls was poisoning their young son. "The dad said we were full of baloney," says McCush. "He wasn't going to stop working."[41]

St. Joseph resident Lauranda Mignery was terrified when, at her son Kadin's one-year doctor visit, his lead levels were so dangerously high that he needed treatment immediately. She had moved into an older home that was affordable for her. No one had told her about the alarming rates of lead poisoning in the neighborhood. After her scare with Kadin's blood lead level, Mignery learned that 20 percent of children in her area who had been tested for lead showed blood levels high enough to be considered lead poisoned.

South Bend, Indiana, was also identified as a problem spot for lead contamination. In one particular census tract, 31 percent of young children had alarmingly high lead levels. One of these children was two-year-old Edward Brown, who as a baby lived with his mother in an older home in central South Bend. When Edward was tested for lead, his blood level was high—90 mcg/dL. Such a massive amount of lead in a small child can be life threatening, provoking seizures or coma. Edward was immediately hospitalized and treated, which reduced his lead levels. His family moved to a newer home, and it seemed that the little boy would beat the odds and get better. He was even meeting many of the typical developmental milestones for a child his age. Still, his mother worries about him. In an interview with Reuters investigators, she expressed her concern, saying: "He's got a lot of energy. Some people think he might have ADHD."[42] As with other children who have been poisoned by lead, only time will tell what effects it may have on Edward.

Poverty Increases Risk

The Reuters investigation revealed a troubling phenomenon that is well known to public health officials and physicians: Low-income communities typically have the worst lead contamination problems in the United States, and their pleas for help are often ignored. "This problem," says Howard Markel, a physician with the University of Michigan School of Public Health, "disproportionately affects the poor—and more specifically, poor African American youngsters—living in our crumbling urban centers." Markel says there is no better example of this than the water crisis in Flint, Michigan, "and the horrific, senseless, and negligent contamination of the

> "This problem disproportionately affects the poor—and more specifically, poor African American youngsters—living in our crumbling urban centers."[43]
>
> —Howard Markel, a physician with the University of Michigan School of Public Health

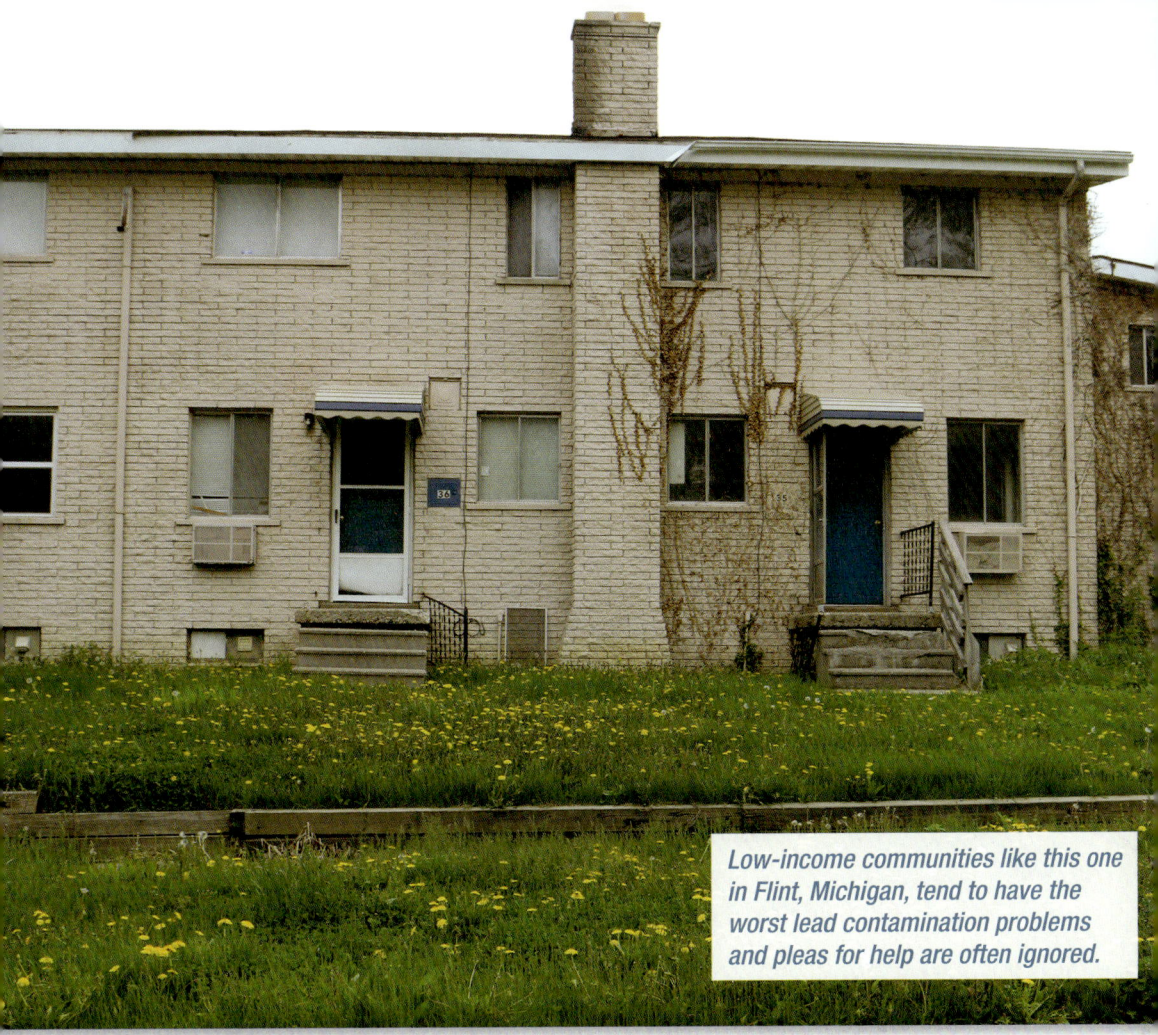

Low-income communities like this one in Flint, Michigan, tend to have the worst lead contamination problems and pleas for help are often ignored.

water supply in this once proud and thriving community."[43] Flint is one of the poorest cities in the United States, with at least 40 percent of residents living below the poverty line. Many people are convinced that what happened there would never have been allowed to happen in a wealthier community.

Throughout the United States, says Markel, thousands of low-income households include children who are being exposed to dangerously high levels of lead. He adds that the landlords who own these aging, low-income homes often neglect to make the necessary repairs because doing so is expensive. The renting parents are struggling to make ends meet and cannot possibly afford to pay for the repairs themselves, nor do they have the financial means to seek safe housing elsewhere. "As a result," says

Markel, "the families living in substandard housing are constantly exposed and re-exposed to this toxin."[44]

In large cities, thousands of people with low incomes live in federally subsidized apartments known as public housing developments. According to the US Department of Housing and Urban Development (HUD), there are approximately 1.3 million units of occupied public housing in the United States. HUD officials estimate that 450,000 of these units were built before 1978 and are therefore likely to have lead paint on the walls and ceilings—which means they are unsafe places for the children who live there. Yet cities are not always conscientious about conducting lead tests in public housing as required by federal law.

Tolanda McMullen lives in a public housing apartment in Chicago, Illinois, that was not inspected for lead before she moved in with her baby boy, Makheil. As he grew, she noticed that Makheil was not hitting the usual milestones for his age group. When he was three, for instance, doctors said he had the language skills of a nine-month-old baby and the cognitive ability of an eighteen-month-old. Blood tests showed that Mikheil's blood lead level was an astronomical 69 mcg/dL. He underwent treatment to rid his body of lead, but the damage was done—and obvious to his mother. "My baby had been healthy," she says. "One day it seemed like the light in his eyes had just gone out."[45]

Lead Dangers in New York's Public Housing

The largest public housing system in the United States is located in New York City, and low-income residents have had a serious, ongoing problem with lead contamination. The New York City Housing Authority, better known as Nycha, oversees 175,000 apartments that collectively house about four hundred thousand people. For years Nycha has been under fire for neglecting its responsibilities to inspect apartments and rid them of lead dangers. New York City law requires that aging public housing units be inspected every year for possible lead paint hazards, but in late 2012 Nycha nonetheless stopped doing inspections. People who

Contaminated Water in Schools

Although no amount of lead is considered safe, the EPA's action level for lead in drinking water is 15 ppb. According to the environmental action group Environment America, lead contamination in the water at schools throughout the United States is much higher than that—and worse than was previously believed. In 2018 the group analyzed water testing results from twenty states and published the findings online in a national interactive map. Problem spots were easily identified, and several states had a large number of school districts with lead-contaminated water.

Some schools had drinking water with an extraordinarily high lead content. One was Leicester Memorial Elementary School in Leicester, Massachusetts, where tap water was found to be 22,400 ppb. In a school in Cleveland, Ohio, water from a drinking fountain tested 1,560 ppb. In suburban areas of Chicago, Illinois, 325 schools do not test for lead, even though testing at 319 other Chicago area schools revealed that 22 percent had lead that exceeded the EPA's standard. One of those tested at more than 3,100 ppm—212 times higher than the EPA action level. "Wherever there are fountains, pipes or plumbing made with lead, there is risk of contamination," says John Rumpler, clean water program director for Environment America. "As more schools test, they are finding this potent neurotoxin in the water our kids drink every day."

Quoted in Environment America, "Lead Contamination in Schools' Drinking Water: Worse than Previously Thought," June 13, 2018. https://environmentamerica.org.

notified the authority about children with elevated blood lead levels were told that Nycha's apartments were not contaminated with lead so the children must have been exposed somewhere else.

This was the case with Mikaila Bonaparte, a little girl who lived in Nycha's Tompkins Houses apartments with her mother. As a toddler, Mikaila crawled around the floor of the apartment, exploring her environment and nibbling on chips of paint that fell from the ceiling and walls. During the summer of 2016, when Mikaila was three years old, she began acting strangely. One minute she seemed lethargic, and then her mood switched to hyperactive. She also cried out as though she were in pain. A blood test showed Mikaila's lead level to be 37 mcg/dL—nearly eight times the CDC's reference level. The city health department sent an inspector, who found high levels of lead in the apartment and ordered Nycha to make repairs. Nycha, in turn, sent its own inspector, who said the apartment did not have an issue with lead paint.

What happened to Mikaila is indicative of a major lead problem throughout New York City's public housing, and this sparked a major investigation of Nycha. One revelation was that from 2010 to 2018, the authority challenged nearly all lead removal orders it received from the health department, just as it had with the findings about Mikaila. The health department, convinced that its initial tests had been false positives, failed to challenge Nycha more than 75 percent of the time.

Over a two-month period in late 2017, city-hired contractors visited eighty-three hundred Nycha apartments and found lead paint contamination in 80 percent of them. In 2018 it was revealed that a total of 1,160 children living in New York City public housing had elevated blood lead levels. The following October New York's mayor vowed that the city would undertake widespread inspections in every public housing unit where lead paint may have been used—more than 140,000 apartments.

Water Unsafe to Drink

Although lead paint is considered the primary source for elevated blood lead levels in children, there are other contributors to the lead problem. As the Flint water crisis showed, an entire city's water supply can be contaminated by lead—with dangerous results. According to the CDC, homes built before 1986 are likely to have lead pipes, lead fixtures, and lead solder. Newer homes, says the agency, may also be at risk if they are built in older neighborhoods. Lead service lines (the pipes that connect the water main in the street to household plumbing systems) in older neighborhoods can leach lead into the water supply. The American Water Works Association estimates that 6.1 million lead service lines are still in operation in the United States, and 22 million Americans are served by those lines. Other potential sources of lead contamination in water include brass fixtures, which often contain lead; galvanized pipes, or pipes that were soldered using lead; and older drinking water coolers that may have lead solder in them.

In April 2018 the *Chicago Tribune* published a report of its investigation of lead contamination in Chicago's water. Nearly three thousand homes in the Chicago area were tested from 2016 to 2018, and high concentrations of lead were found in water drawn from nearly 70 percent of them. In three out of every ten homes sampled, tap water had lead concentrations above 5 parts per billion (ppb), which is the maximum allowed by the US Food and Drug Administration for bottled water. Investigators determined the culprit to be old lead service lines that connect street mains with homes, many of which have not been replaced. Chicago resident Bianca Baker, who had her water tested, says she fears that what happened in Flint could happen in her city. "Anytime you are talking about water," says Baker, "you are talking about life."[46]

> "Anytime you are talking about water, you are talking about life."[46]
>
> —Bianca Baker, a resident of Chicago, Illinois, who worries about lead in the water

Twenty-First-Century Lead Contamination

The lead contamination people hear most about is often called legacy lead: old, crumbling lead paint, lead in the soil from years of industry and automobiles burning leaded gas, and antiquated pipes that allow lead to leach into water supplies. Although these sources collectively represent the most serious lead dangers in the United States, not all lead contamination is related to polluting practices from the past. Lead is still being emitted into the atmosphere, and it is contributing to the country's lead contamination problem.

For instance, motor vehicles can no longer burn leaded gas, but the law that banned it did not end the use of leaded gas altogether. Lead-containing fuel known as aviation gasoline (avgas) is still burned by piston-engine aircraft, which include small propeller-driven planes, seaplanes, and some helicopters. According to the Federal Aviation Administration (FAA), there are more than 167,000 of these aircraft operating in the United States. Collectively, avgas-burning aircraft emit more than 450 tons (408.2 metric tons) of lead into the atmosphere each year and represent the country's largest source of lead emissions.

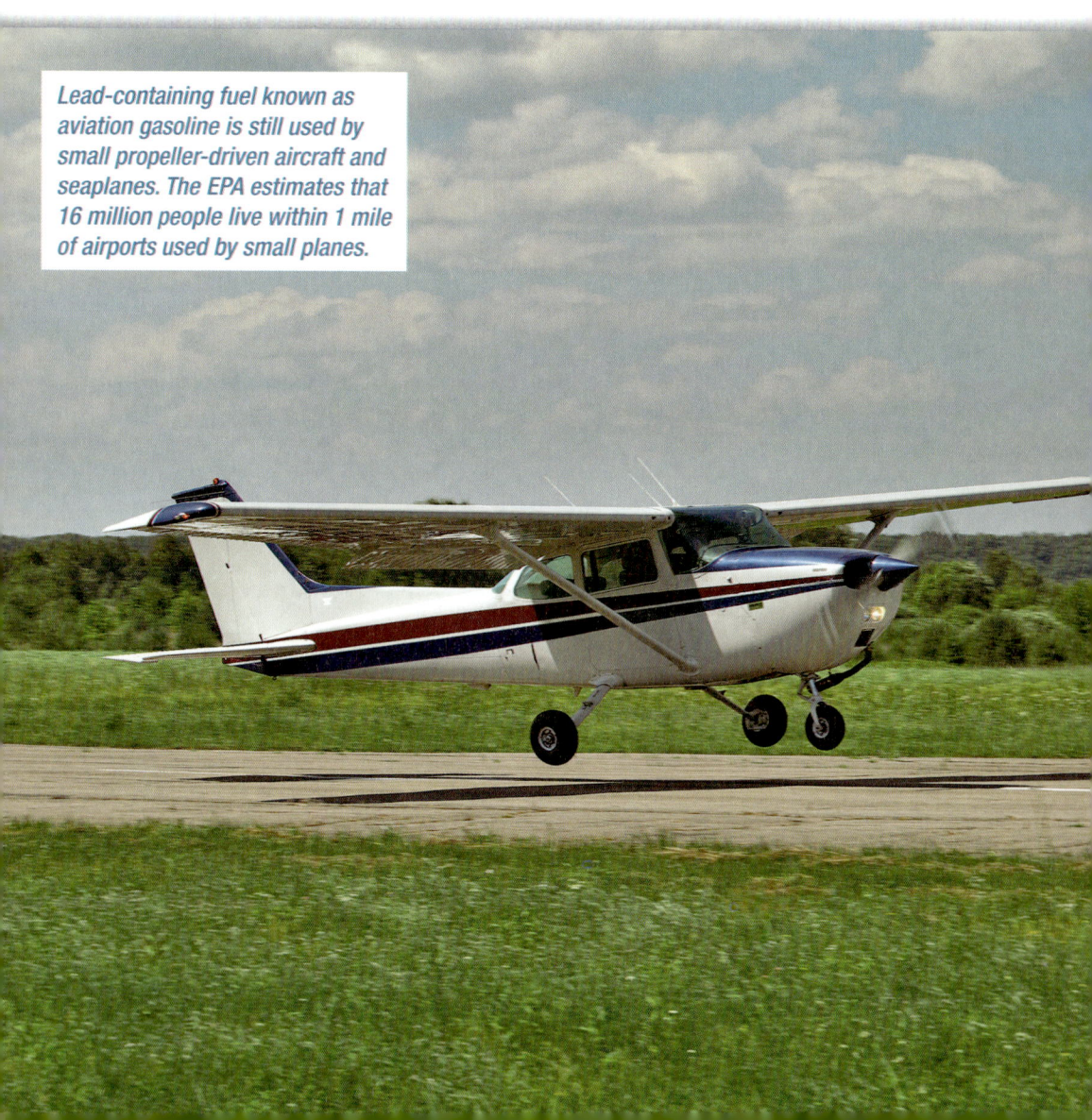

Lead-containing fuel known as aviation gasoline is still used by small propeller-driven aircraft and seaplanes. The EPA estimates that 16 million people live within 1 mile of airports used by small planes.

The Connection Between Lead and Crime

As serious as lead contamination is in the United States, years of declining lead in the atmosphere has made a positive difference. Whereas leaded gasoline once filled the air with lead particles, for more than twenty years the fuel has been banned for use in automobiles. People undoubtedly know this has enabled them to breathe cleaner air, but they may not be aware that it could also have helped reduce crime. According to a theory known as the lead-crime hypothesis, that is exactly what happened.

The theory originated with researchers who studied a mysterious drop in crime during the 1990s, after extraordinarily high crime rates during the 1970s and 1980s. The researchers drew a clear connection between the rise and fall of crime and the rise and fall of lead in the atmosphere. Specifically, when the use of leaded gasoline was widespread, the crime rate skyrocketed. When leaded gas was phasing out, crime began to drop. Journalist Kevin Drum, who is known for his research of the lead-crime connection, writes:

> By 2010, an entire generation of teenagers and young adults—the age group responsible for the most crime—had grown up nearly lead free, and the violent crime rate had plummeted to half or less of its high point. This happened across the board: in big and small cities; among blacks and whites; in every state; in every city; and, as it turns out, in every other country that also phased out leaded gasoline.

Kevin Drum, "An Updated Lead-Crime Roundup for 2018," *Mother Jones*, February 1, 2018. www.motherjones.com.

The EPA estimates that 16 million people, including 3 million children, live or attend school within 1 mile (1.6 km) of airports with aircraft that burn avgas. Research has shown that children who live close to these airports have higher blood lead levels than children living farther away. No regulatory action has been taken to discontinue the use of avgas, although the FAA and EPA have had long-term discussions about phasing it out. For environmentalists

> "In light of the evidence and the lives hanging in the balance, EPA must cease stalling and quickly move to regulate and ultimately eliminate the threat of lead poisoning from avgas."[47]
>
> —Miki Barnes, president of the public interest group Oregon Aviation Watch

and watchdog groups, that cannot happen soon enough. "The facts are clear," says Miki Barnes, president of the public interest group Oregon Aviation Watch. "There is no 'safe' level of blood lead, or exposure to lead, especially for children. That's why the law protects us from lead in paint and in our automobiles. In light of the evidence and the lives hanging in the balance, EPA must cease stalling and quickly move to regulate and ultimately eliminate the threat of lead poisoning from avgas as well."[47]

A Seemingly Endless Problem

Lead contamination in the United States has lessened over the years, but that does not mean the problem no longer exists. Cities throughout the country are plagued by the dangers of old lead paint in apartments and houses, and this puts children's health at risk. Water contaminated by lead is not as common as lead paint, but it is still a problem for Americans in many cities. As people begin to understand that lead contamination is not as rare as they may have believed, this may result in lasting change. Until that happens, the public—especially young children—will continue to be threatened by the dangers of lead.

CHAPTER FOUR

An Urgent Search for Solutions

Scientific evidence leaves no doubt that lead is a dangerous substance that causes severe, permanent health damage, especially to young children. There is also plenty of evidence that despite reductions in children's blood lead levels in the past two decades, lead contamination is still a formidable problem; the only safe amount of lead is no lead. Yet even though these facts have been firmly established and verified, the United States lacks any nationwide effort to clean up legacy lead, put an end to new lead contamination, and prevent children and adults from being exposed to and harmed by lead. In the August 2017 issue of *Harvard Environmental Law Review*, Emily A. Benfer, founding director of the Health Justice Project and clinical professor of law at Loyola University of Chicago, published a scathing assessment of America's failure to address its widespread lead problem. She writes:

> Rather than identifying and controlling the lead hazard before a child is harmed, public policy follows a predominantly "wait and see" approach. For example, the majority of local, state, and federal programs require that a child develop lead poisoning before lead hazard investigation and remediation in the child's environment is permitted or required. These lead poisoning "prevention" policies are hardly preventative in nature, create a false sense of safety, and mislead the public.[48]

Prevention Must Be the Focus

Benfer's strong objections to the wait-and-see approach are overwhelmingly shared by pediatricians, researchers, and others who are knowledgeable about the dangers of lead. Pediatrician Bruce P. Lanphear is an expert who is adamant about the urgency of prevention efforts, as he writes: "The primary prevention approach contrasts with practices and policies that too often have relied predominantly on detection of lead exposure only after children develop elevated blood lead concentrations."[49] Lanphear emphasizes that the key to preventing lead poisoning in children is identification and elimination of the major sources of exposure: lead paint in older housing, lead-contaminated soil, and lead in public water supplies.

Two like-minded experts are Philip Landrigan and David Bellinger. Landrigan, a pediatrician and the first to document the effects of lead poisoning in American children, and Bellinger, a Harvard Medical School professor of neurology, refer to lead as a "devastating poison" and to America's lead exposure problem as an "epidemic."[50] They find the idea of addressing lead contamination with a wait-and-see approach, as described by Benfer, to be unconscionable, and they compare it to a practice that was once used by coal miners in Britain and the United States.

While working in an underground mine, the miners needed to monitor the air for dangerous buildups of carbon monoxide and other poisonous gases. So they kept a caged canary with them in the mine. If the bird became ill or died, the miners knew they had to evacuate. "We seem to use children in the same way to warn us of lead," Landrigan and Bellinger write. "We wait for a child to become poisoned before we investigate the source of exposure. Given the limited options for treating children with lead poisoning,

> "Rather than identifying and controlling the lead hazard before a child is harmed, public policy follows a predominantly 'wait and see' approach."[48]
>
> —Emily A. Benfer, founding director of the Health Justice Project and clinical professor of law at Loyola University of Chicago

this is poor public health and bad medicine. We need to identify lead hazards before they harm children."[51]

Three Essential Phases

Landrigan and Bellinger emphasize that to address the problem of lead contamination and lead poisoning among children, a comprehensive plan is needed. The first step is mapping the sources of lead throughout the United States and then using the findings to create a national map of problem areas. "In this era of big

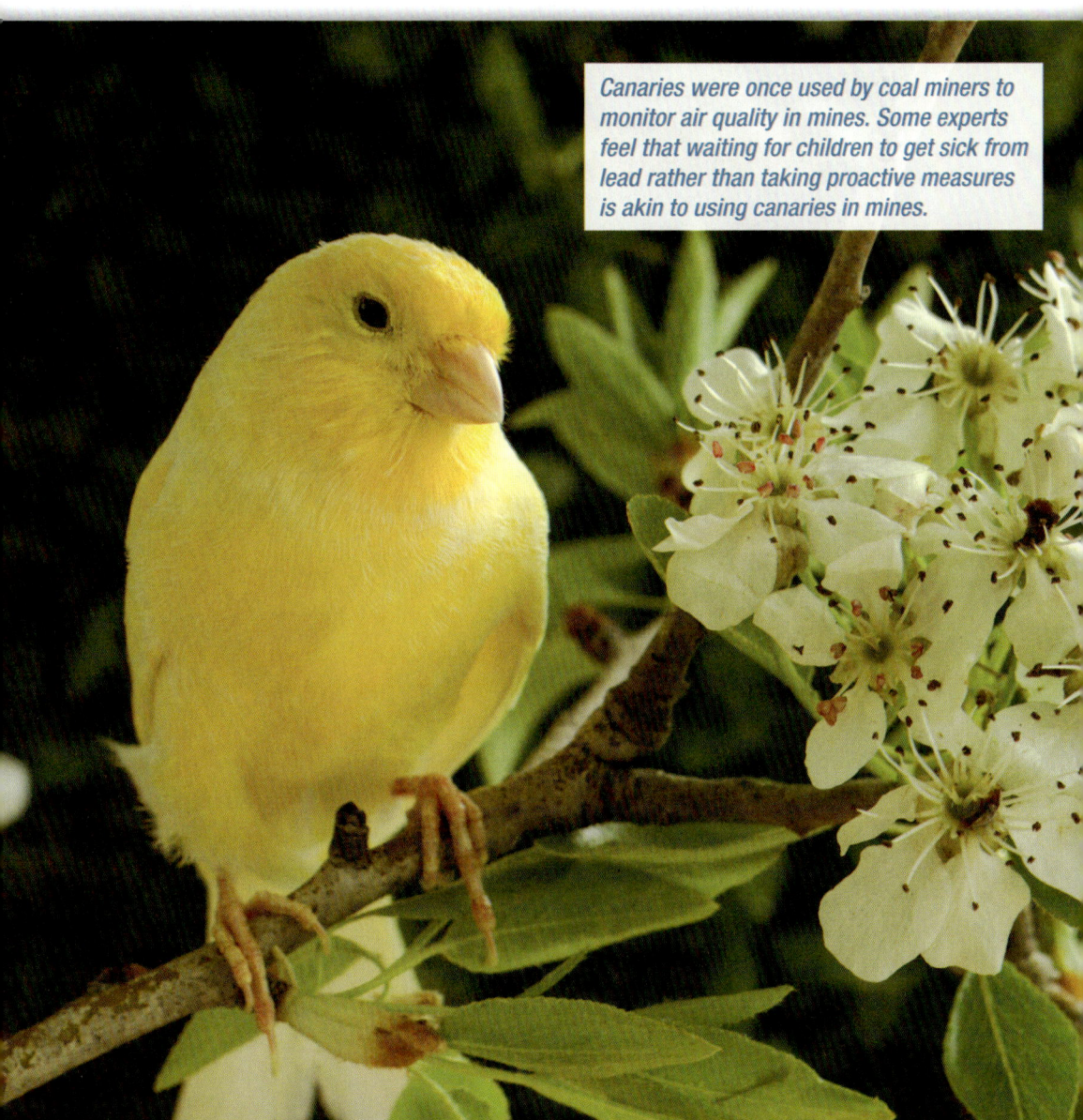

Canaries were once used by coal miners to monitor air quality in mines. Some experts feel that waiting for children to get sick from lead rather than taking proactive measures is akin to using canaries in mines.

data when we can monitor billions of telephone conversations and visualize traces of water on Pluto," they write, "it is incomprehensible that we do not have a fine-grained national map of the sources of lead in America."[52]

The second part of the plan they envision involves containing and reducing lead that was identified in the mapping phase. This would be a large and complex undertaking that would involve removing lead paint from homes, replacing lead pipes and service lines, and cleaning up contaminated soils. Yet Landrigan and Bellinger are convinced that the effort would pay for itself over time. "These actions are highly cost-effective because they

---

The Gift of Clean Water

Flint is one of the poorest cities in the United States, with more than half of its children living in poverty. After the water crisis, residents had no idea when or even whether they would have clean, safe water in their homes and schools, and this was a frightening uncertainty. Fortunately, all the old underground lead pipes are being replaced with new copper piping—more than eighteen thousand pipes in all, with the work to be completed sometime in 2020. The schools, however, needed new water filtration systems, and this was a financial burden for the cash-strapped city. Then the school district heard from a billionaire named Elon Musk, the founder of Tesla and SpaceX, saying that he wanted to help—and help he did.

In August 2018 officials from Flint Community Schools announced that Musk had donated nearly $500,000 for the purchase and installation of new water systems for all twelve Flint schools and the administration building. The high-tech systems disinfect and filter out all lead and bacteria from the water, which will provide students at all the schools with sparkling-clean water from fountains. Flint superintendent of schools Derrick Lopez says everyone is "deeply grateful" to Musk and that the new system will help students "return to the normalcy of what should be a fundamental right: having access to safe, clean water."

Quoted in Roberto Acosta, "Elon Musk Donates $480K to Flint Schools for UV Water Filtration Systems," MLive, October 5, 2018. www.mlive.com.

prevent disease and lifelong disability not only in today's children, but in all future generations," they write. The third and final phase of the program is to "make sure there is no new lead." Landrigan and Bellinger urge policy makers to take steps to eliminate all nonessential uses of lead, such as replacing lead-acid batteries with lead-free technology. "Now is the time to end the profound immorality of lead poisoning in America," they write. "We have the science. We know how to do the job. What we need is leadership, courage and political will."[53]

> "Now is the time to end the profound immorality of lead poisoning in America."[53]
>
> —Philip Landrigan, a pediatrician and noted lead expert, and David Bellinger, professor of neurology at Harvard Medical School

A Proactive City

In the absence of a comprehensive nationwide plan for addressing lead contamination, many localities are putting their own measures in place. One of them is Cleveland, Ohio, a midwestern city where exposure to old lead paint has caused severe problems for young children. According to the Ohio Department of Health, from 2016 to 2017 about 12 percent of Cleveland children who were screened for lead tested above the CDC's 5 mcg/dL reference level and required medical attention. This is significantly higher than the national average of 3 percent, so health officials knew an action plan was needed.

In September 2018 Cleveland city officials partnered with the school district, nonprofit organizations, and Case Western Reserve University to implement the Partners in Health Lead Screening Program. It is unique because children are tested at school, rather than parents having to seek out testing on their own, which often results in no testing. Surveys have shown that even though Ohio requires lead testing for young children covered by Medicaid, only about one-third of the at-risk children living in Cleveland are ever tested. The school program is intended to make it easier for parents to get their children tested for lead, and to test children at a young age before they show any symptoms of lead poisoning.

The program, which kicked off at the beginning of the 2018–2019 school year, is supervised by two longtime nurses, Lynn Lotas and Debbie Aloshen. At about thirty different schools, student nurses and community volunteers prick the fingers of children three to five years old to get a drop of blood that is tested for lead. Children who are found to have lead blood levels of 5 mcg/dL or more receive follow-up care. The idea, says Aloshen, is to focus on prevention—finding children who have a risk of being harmed by lead exposure and getting them help before that happens. "What we think we can do is get a better handle of which kids have a problem, which neighborhoods are worse than others, and get treatment started earlier,"[54] she says.

The program in Cleveland also involves information sharing, which is a crucial aspect of helping kids affected by lead exposure. Data obtained through the blood tests will be shared with city, county, and federal agencies to determine the best programs and policies for the children found to have high blood lead levels. City officials hope that this information sharing will help identify high-risk areas for lead exposure from old lead paint. In Cleveland these will likely include inner-city areas, which have a high poverty rate and many old houses and apartments, as well as the sites of former industries whose lead-filled emissions polluted the soil. "I don't know of any other cities in the country testing at schools like this," says public health physician Giridhar Mallya, "and it will likely turn out to be a good way to increase the rate at which young children are getting tested."[55] Mallya and other supporters of Cleveland's program hope that other cities and states will protect vulnerable children by putting their own similar programs in place.

A Massive Undertaking in Michigan

Michigan is one state that has done exactly that. As a direct result of the Flint water crisis and state government officials being held accountable for their egregious mishandling of it, Michigan

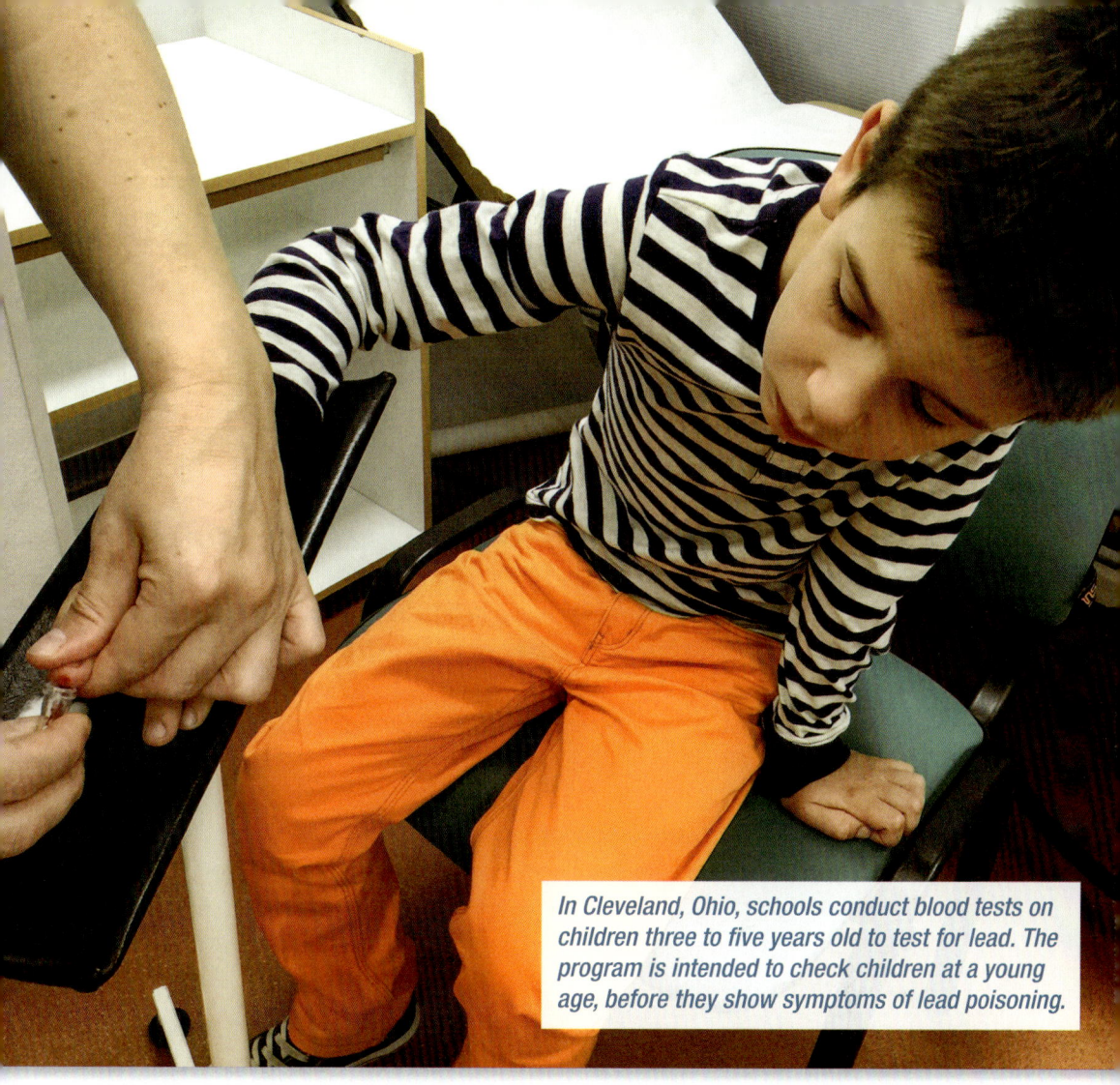

In Cleveland, Ohio, schools conduct blood tests on children three to five years old to test for lead. The program is intended to check children at a young age, before they show symptoms of lead poisoning.

enacted sweeping new regulations that are some of the strictest in the United States. These new policies were announced in June 2018 and involve the replacement of all Michigan's lead service lines that carry drinking water—about five hundred thousand of them. This massive project will begin no later than 2021 and is expected to take about twenty years to complete. "These new protections can never make up for the disaster in Flint," says Cyndi Roper, Natural Resources Defense Council senior policy advocate. "And while they don't solve the whole problem, they help ensure that other communities are better protected moving forward."[56]

> ## A Cautionary Report
>
> For people concerned about lead in water from their home plumbing systems, the CDC recommends they run cold water through the tap for one to two minutes, which is supposed to help flush out lead. But according to July 2018 research from LSU Health in New Orleans, Louisiana, this technique is not consistently effective—and sometimes it does not help at all.
>
> From February 2015 to November 2016, the researchers surveyed home owners and tested water samples from 376 New Orleans homes on the East Bank of the Mississippi River (the city's water source). The samples were drawn from tap water that had been running for three different intervals: thirty to forty-five seconds, two and a half to three minutes, and five and a half to six minutes. Nearly all samples were found to contain some lead, although levels far below the EPA's action point of 15 ppb. In testing samples drawn for the various times, there was no significant difference in lead levels until the six-minute mark, after which lead did decrease. From this the researchers concluded that the CDC's recommendation for flushing a water system does not necessarily protect children from lead in drinking water. "More effective interventions like certified water filters should be considered instead," says lead researcher Adrienne Katner, "particularly when replacing water service lines and plumbing is not economically possible."
>
> Quoted in Leslie Capo, "Study Finds Flushing Water Lines Protects Inconsistently and May Increase Lead Exposure," LSU Health, July 23, 2018. www.lsuhsc.edu.

In addition to the replacement of the state's lead service lines, Michigan has also lowered its action level for lead content in drinking water. Whereas the CDC recommends the maximum lead content to be 15 ppb, the Michigan limit will be 12 ppb. Although these new regulations cover only lead-contaminated risks to water—and some critics say they do not go far enough—environmental advocates hailed the state's action, saying it was a long time coming. In the opinion of Natural Resources Defense Council senior director Eric Olson, Michigan has taken action that will potentially set an example for others. "A lot of other states have been wrestling with this question, [but] not a lot of them have stepped up to adopt or propose a rule like Michigan's," says Olson. "We're hoping Michigan adopting this will spur other states to step up."[57]

Other states have started to address problems with lead contamination, although Olson says their slow progress is frustrating. "I wouldn't say I'm getting goosebumps about how fast they are,"[58] he says. Still, he and other environmental advocates acknowledge that even slow progress is better than no progress, especially in the absence of an action plan by the federal government.

New Hampshire Takes Action

Like Michigan, New Hampshire has also enacted tough new legislation. With some of the oldest housing in the entire country, New Hampshire has struggled with the effects of lead paint. It is everywhere, and it presents a formidable and alarming health risk for the state's children. Each year, several hundred children are diagnosed with lead poisoning. In 2016, for instance, 741 children tested had blood lead levels either at or above the CDC's 5 mcg/dL level of concern, which was nearly a 17 percent increase over 2015, when 634 children tested that high. Health officials fear that the actual number is much higher, since not all children are tested. With new legislation signed into law in February 2018, more at-risk children will likely be identified.

According to Tom Irwin, a New Hampshire resident who directs the Conservation Law Foundation, the state's new law strengthens existing lead laws in several important ways. One is that New Hampshire will become one of the states that requires universal testing, meaning that all one- and two-year-old children will be tested for lead, with the costs covered by insurance. "This important change will dramatically increase the number of kids currently being tested for lead poisoning," says Irwin, "ensuring better protection for many more children."[59] Another part of the new law is lowering the reference level of blood lead content in children to 5 mcg/dL by 2021. This is consistent with the CDC's recommendation and much lower than New Hampshire's previous reference level of 10 mcg/dL.

Another aspect of New Hampshire's new law is requirements to address potential exposure to lead in drinking water. Schools and child care facilities will be required to test their water and undertake corrective action if lead is found to be above the EPA standard of 15 ppb. Also, the law requires the state to notify parents and landlords if a child is found to have a blood lead level of 3 mcg/dL. And if property owners need to eliminate hazards from old lead paint, they can obtain guaranteed loans from a state program. Irwin calls the law a "major, much-needed step forward in addressing the ongoing problem of childhood lead poisoning." Although it is not perfect and there is a great deal of work to be done, he says, "It goes without saying that the health of our kids is worth it."[60]

Publicity Spurs Action on Military Bases

As cities and states enact measures to help protect children from lead exposure, the US military has undertaken its own corrective action—but rather than being proactive, the efforts followed an investigation that triggered public outrage. The investigation was conducted during 2018 by reporters from Reuters. It revealed that children living on military bases were being exposed to lead paint in their homes and nothing was being done to prevent it. According to investigative reporters Joshua Schneyer and Andrea Januta, it is a US Army requirement that if testing identifies deteriorating lead paint in base homes, repairs must be made. The investigation found, however, that army officials discourage lead inspections because repairs can be so expensive. Schneyer and Januta write, "These homes put military kids at risk."[61] Another revelation was that more than one thousand children living on US

> "These homes put military kids at risk."[61]
>
> —Reuters investigative reporters Joshua Schneyer and Andrea Januta

Army bases tested high for blood lead concentrations in recent years. But army clinics that performed the test often failed to report high test results to state health authorities as required.

The investigative report was released in August 2018. Within a week, military officials announced that major corrective action would be taken. The army plans to test forty thousand older homes for lead and, whenever necessary, to remove and relocate families from the homes. The effort is expected to cost as much as $386 million to complete. For Karla Hughes, who lives with her army captain husband and four-year-old daughter at the military base in Fort Knox, Kentucky, this renewed attention to lead contamination on the part of military officials is a welcome change. Hughes discovered old lead paint on many occasions around the base and on her own front porch, but when she complained, she was told that there was no problem. Without the Reuters investigation, she says, "this danger may have been left undiscovered and ignored."[62]

Researchers Reach Out

One of the most crucial elements of any lead-prevention program is testing, yet research has shown that widespread testing is rare in the United States. This is true whether the testing is to determine lead content in soil, the existence of lead paint in houses and apartments, or lead content in drinking water. Researchers and students from Princeton University are trying to make a positive difference in Trenton, New Jersey, by conducting water testing at no charge to residents. The program, which combines environmental science with community service, is called the Urban Tap Water and Human Health project.

Princeton students, supervised by professors John Higgins and Janet Currie, use cutting-edge technology to gather water samples around Trenton. Then back in the school laboratory, they analyze the samples. As of November 2017 the students had analyzed about 750 water samples from 245 Trenton households.

They found the average lead content to be 2.5 ppb, with only a small percentage of the homes tested exceeding the CDC's action level of 15 ppb. The technology they use for analysis is highly sophisticated and allows them to pinpoint where lead in drinking water is coming from, such as from a water main or a home's plumbing. For instance, the presence of metals like cadmium and zinc may indicate that the contamination is caused by lead solder or pipe fittings. "You need fairly complicated instruments to do these measurements well—it's not common overall," says Hig-

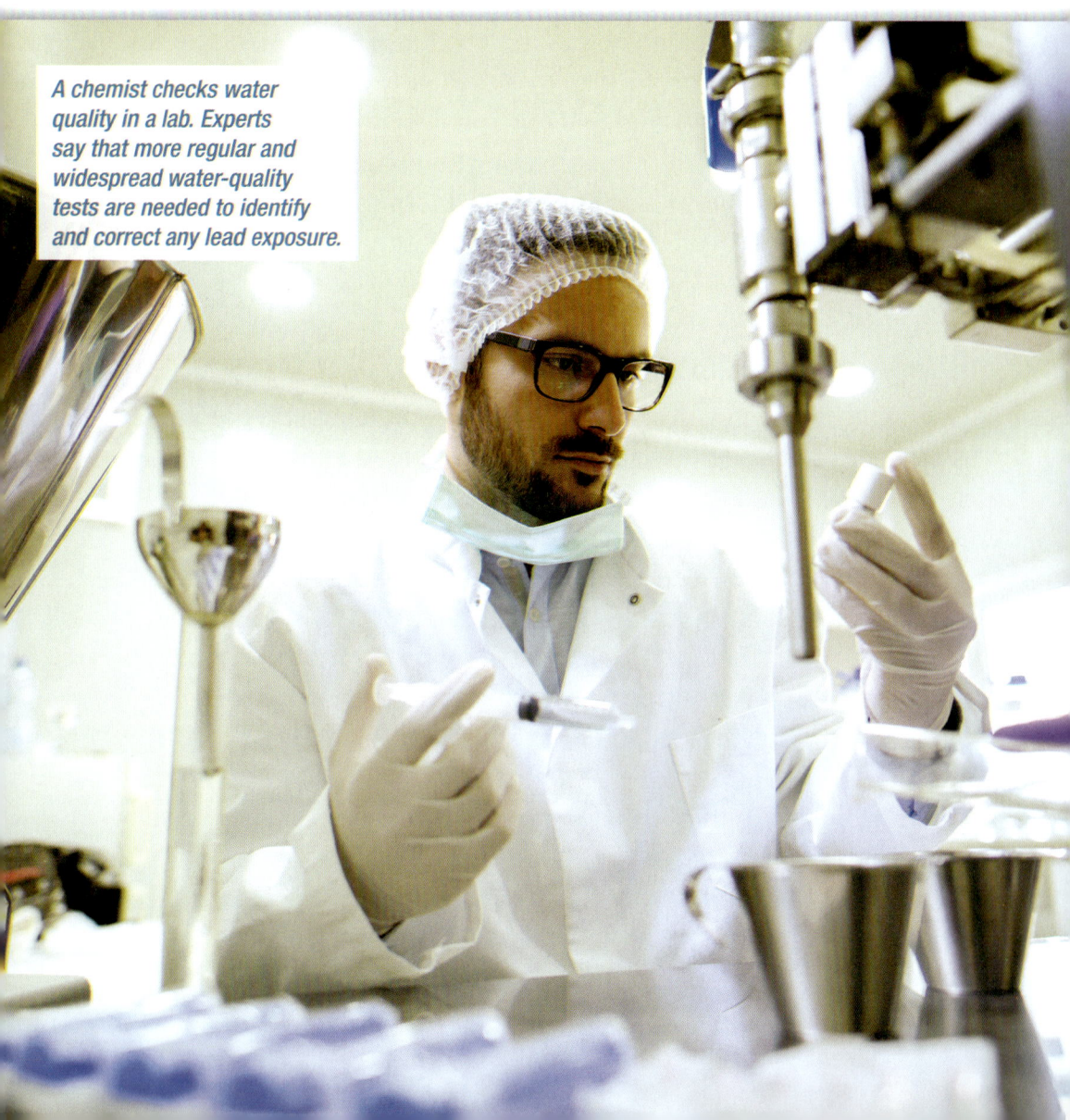

A chemist checks water quality in a lab. Experts say that more regular and widespread water-quality tests are needed to identify and correct any lead exposure.

gins. "It's about being able to put your finger on what the source of the contamination is."[63]

College students at Indiana University–Purdue University Indianapolis (IUPUI) are also participating in lead testing with their earth science professor, Gabriel Filippelli, whose research has focused on lead contamination in soil. He requests that people throughout the United States and Canada provide him with samples of the dust in their homes, which they can do by vacuuming and then sending the dust in a plastic bag. Filippelli and his students analyze the dust for various contaminants. They generate a report from their findings and send it back to the residents, along with instructions for how to avoid any health risks associated with the contaminants.

Filippelli emphasizes that lead inside people's homes is not always from old lead paint on the interior walls. It can also result from lead that gets in the soil due to old crumbling exterior paint, the remains of old industry, or all the years when leaded gas was burned in automobiles. Once this contamination is in the soil, it can be tracked in on people's shoes. "Dirt outside doesn't just stay outside," says Filippelli. "If the soil is high [in lead], it's likely that some of that goes inside homes."[64] He adds that people who want to know more about lead contamination in their homes have few options available. He is trying to fill that gap by making it easy for them to get needed testing done.

> "Dirt outside doesn't just stay outside. If the soil is high [in lead], it's likely that some of that goes inside homes."[64]
>
> —Gabriel Filippelli, professor of earth sciences at IUPUI

An Extraordinarily Tough Problem to Solve

Few people would disagree that the United States has a lead contamination problem. And if they do, there is plenty of evidence to convince them otherwise. What is far more difficult to establish, however, is exactly what should be done to fix the problem. The federal government, which in the past saw the need for laws to protect people from lead, seems to have adopted a hands-off approach, leaving it up to states and cities to put their own measures in place and supporting them with federal dollars when warranted. But experts say this is not enough, that much more needs to be done because children's health—and their futures—depend on it. What happened in Flint has triggered numerous lead exposure prevention programs, not only in Michigan but other states and cities as well. Perhaps that crisis, as devastating as it was, will prove to be a catalyst for much-needed change.

SOURCE NOTES

Introduction: Dangerous Metal

1. Mona Hanna-Attisha, "Opinion: How a Pediatrician Became a Detective," *New York Times*, June 9, 2018. www.nytimes.com.
2. Quoted in Plinio Prioreschi, *A History of Medicine: Roman Medicine*. Omaha, NE: Horatius, 1998, p. 279.
3. Fiona E. McNeill, "From IQ to Blood Pressure, We Should Not Be Complacent About Lead," The Conversation, April 3, 2018. https://theconversation.com.
4. Quoted in Cleveland Clinic, "Why Lead Is Dangerous for Your Child—and Its Surprising Sources," January 22, 2016. https://health.clevelandclinic.org.

Chapter One: Public Health Crises in the Making

5. Quoted in Lynne Peeples, "Lead Paint Trial: Did Industry Promote Product Knowing of Its Toxic Dangers?," *Huffington Post*, December 6, 2017. www.huffingtonpost.com.
6. Quoted in Regina Cole, "The State's Battle with Lead Paint Is Far from Won," *Boston Globe*, August 17, 2016. www.bostonglobe.com.
7. Michael Collins, "Big EPA Fines for Violating 'Little' Lead Paint Rule," GLE Associates, 2016. www.gleassociates.com.
8. Quoted in Meredith Parker, "1 in 6 Children in Savannah's Historic District Living with High Lead Levels," WTOC, February 6, 2018. www.wtoc.com.
9. Quoted in Rick Montgomery, "It's Been 40 Years Since Lead Paint Was Banned, So Why Are We Still Being Poisoned?," *Kansas City (MO) Star*, March 23, 2018. www.kansascity.com.
10. Quoted in Sydney Pereira, "Private Buildings Have a Load of Lead Problems, Too: Tenants, Advocates," *Villager* (Manhattan), September 23, 2018. http://thevillager.com.

11. Quoted in Christine MacDonald, "Detroit to Halt Some Demolitions over Lead Concerns," *Detroit (MI) News*, March 20, 2018. www.detroitnews.com.
12. Quoted in Nicole C. Brambila, "Coming Clean: EPA Cleaned Lead-Contaminated Soil at Muhlenberg Personal Care Home," *Reading (PA) Eagle*, September 24, 2018. www.readingeagle.com.
13. Quoted in Darwin BondGraham, "Oakland's Toxic Lead Contamination Isn't in the Water. It's in the Buildings and Dirt, and It's Bad," *East Bay Express* (Oakland, CA), December 29, 2016. www.eastbayexpress.com.
14. Quoted in CBS News, "In Philadelphia, High Levels of Lead in Soil Raise Parents' Concerns," October 9, 2017. www.cbsnews.com.
15. Barbara Laker et al., "In Booming Philly Neighborhoods, Lead-Poisoned Soil Is Resurfacing," *Philadelphia Inquirer*, June 18, 2017. www.philly.com.
16. Quoted in Lake et al., "In Booming Philly Neighborhoods, Lead-Poisoned Soil Is Resurfacing."
17. Quoted in Liz Leyden, "In Echo of Flint, Mich., Water Crisis Now Hits Newark," *New York Times*, October 30, 2018. www.nytimes.com.
18. Quoted in Leyden, "In Echo of Flint, Mich., Water Crisis Now Hits Newark."
19. Quoted in Leyden, "In Echo of Flint, Mich., Water Crisis Now Hits Newark."
20. US Environmental Protection Agency, "A Public Health Approach to Addressing Lead," January 10, 2017. www.epa.gov.

Chapter Two: A Heavy Toll on Human Health

21. Mary Gearing, "The Deadly Biology of Lead Exposure," Science in the News, Harvard University, June 27, 2016. http://sitn.hms.harvard.edu.
22. Gearing, "The Deadly Biology of Lead Exposure."

23. Gearing, "The Deadly Biology of Lead Exposure."
24. Quoted in Ben Tinker, "Why Lead Is So Dangerous for Children," CNN, January 29, 2016. www.cnn.com.
25. Bruce P. Lanphear, "The Impact of Toxins on the Developing Brain," *Annual Review of Public Health*, March 2015. www.annualreviews.org.
26. Quoted in Kristen Jordan Shamus, "What Every Parent Needs to Know About Lead Poisoning," *Detroit (MI) Free Press*, February 13, 2016. www.freep.com.
27. Howard Markel, "How a Doctor Discovered U.S. Walls Were Poisonous," *PBS NewsHour*, March 29, 2013. www.pbs.org.
28. Quoted in Terrence McCoy, "Washington's Worst Case of Lead Poisoning in Decades Happened in a Home Sanctioned by Housing Officials," *Washington Post*, January 30, 2017. www.washingtonpost.com.
29. Daniel S. Grossman and David J.G. Slusky, "The Effect of an Increase in Lead in the Water System on Fertility and Birth Outcomes: The Case of Flint, Michigan," University of Kansas, August 7, 2017. www2.ku.edu.
30. Stefano Renzetti et al., "The Association of Lead Exposure During Pregnancy and Childhood Anthropometry in the Mexican PROGRESS Cohort," *Environmental Research*, January 2017. www.ncbi.nlm.nih.gov.
31. Quoted in Tinker, "Why Lead Is So Dangerous for Children."
32. Quoted in Emily Atkin, "Did Flint's Water Crisis Damage Kids' Brains?," *New Republic*, February 14, 2018. https://newrepublic.com.
33. Quoted in Joshua Schneyer and Andrea Januta, "Children Poisoned by Lead on U.S. Army Bases as Hazards Go Ignored," Reuters, August 16, 2018. www.reuters.com.
34. Quoted in Schneyer and Januta, "Children Poisoned by Lead on U.S. Army Bases as Hazards Go Ignored."
35. Quoted in Alexandra Ossola, "Lead in Water: What Are the Health Effects and Dangers?," *Popular Science*, January 18, 2016. www.popsci.com.

Chapter Three: No End in Sight

36. Marc Edwards, "Experiences and Observations from the 2001–2004 'DC Lead Crisis,'" Virginia Tech, May 17, 2010. http://flintwaterstudy.org.
37. Edwards, "Experiences and Observations from the 2001–2004 'DC Lead Crisis.'"
38. Joshua Schneyer and M.B. Pell, "Millions of American Children Missing Early Lead Tests, Reuters Finds," Reuters, June 9, 2016. www.reuters.com.
39. M.B. Pell and Joshua Schneyer, "Special Report: Thousands of U.S. Areas Afflicted with Lead Poisoning Beyond Flint's," Reuters, December 19, 2016. www.reuters.com.
40. Quoted in Pell and Schneyer, "Special Report."
41. Quoted in Pell and Schneyer, "Special Report."
42. Quoted in Pell and Schneyer, "Special Report."
43. Howard Markel, "Remember Flint," *Milbank Quarterly*, June 2016. www.ncbi.nlm.nih.gov.
44. Markel, "Remember Flint."
45. Quoted in Michael Hawthorne and Jennifer Smith Richards, "Kids Poisoned by Lead in CHA Housing; Landlords Still Got Paid," *Chicago Tribune*, April 8, 2017. www.chicagotribune.com.
46. Quoted in Michael Hawthorne, "Flint Researchers Find Alarming Levels of Lead in Cicero, Berwyn Tap Water, Suggesting Thousands of Older Homes at Risk," *Chicago Tribune*, August 10, 2018. www.chicagotribune.com.
47. Quoted in Friends of the Earth, "Groups Press EPA to Address Toxic Lead Air Pollution from Aviation Gasoline," April 2014. https://foe.org.

Chapter Four: An Urgent Search for Solutions

48. Emily A. Benfer, "Contaminated Childhood: How the United States Failed to Prevent the Chronic Lead Poisoning of Low-Income Children and Communities of Color," *Harvard Environmental Law Review*, August 2017. http://harvardelr.com.
49. Bruce P. Lanphear, "Prevention of Childhood Lead Toxicity," *Pediatrics*, July 2016. http://pediatrics.aappublications.org.

50. Philip Landrigan and David Bellinger, "How to Finally End Lead Poisoning in America," *Time*, April 11, 2016. http://time.com.
51. Landrigan and Bellinger, "How to Finally End Lead Poisoning in America."
52. Landrigan and Bellinger, "How to Finally End Lead Poisoning in America."
53. Landrigan and Bellinger, "How to Finally End Lead Poisoning in America."
54. Quoted in Daniel McGraw, "A New Test in Cleveland's Schools," *US News & World Report*, September 13, 2018. www.usnews.com.
55. Quoted in McGraw, "A New Test in Cleveland's Schools."
56. Quoted in David Eggert, "Michigan Now Has Nation's Toughest Rules for Lead in Drinking Water," *Detroit (MI) Free Press*, June 14, 2018. www.freep.com.
57. Quoted in E.A. Crunden, "Michigan's Sweeping New Water Regulations Set New Standard for States Plagued by Lead," ThinkProgress, June 18, 2018. https://thinkprogress.org.
58. Quoted in Eggert, "Michigan Now Has Nation's Toughest Rules for Lead in Drinking Water."
59. Tom Irwin, "New Hampshire Kids Now Better Protected from Lead Poisoning," Conservation Law Foundation, February 9, 2018. www.clf.org.
60. Irwin, "New Hampshire Kids Now Better Protected from Lead Poisoning."
61. Schneyer and Januta, "Children Poisoned on U.S. Army Bases as Hazards Go Ignored."
62. Quoted in Joshua Schneyer, "Special Report: Reuters' Testing Triggers Lead Cleanup at Fort Knox Base," *U.S. News & World Report*, August 16, 2018. www.usnews.com.
63. Quoted in Morgan Kelly, "Studying Lead Contamination in Trenton, N.J.," Princeton University, April 2, 2018. www.princeton.edu.
64. Quoted in Emily Hopkins, "The Dust in Your Home Could Be Contaminated with Lead. This Researcher Wants to Help You," *IndyStar*, July 15, 2018. www.indystar.com.

ORGANIZATIONS AND WEBSITES

American Public Health Association
800 Eye St. NW
Washington, DC 20001
website: www.apha.org

The American Public Health Association seeks to improve the health of the public and achieve equity in health status. A number of publications about lead contamination, lead exposure, the health hazards of lead, and other related topics are available on its website.

Centers for Disease Control and Prevention (CDC)
Lead Poisoning Prevention Program
1600 Clifton Rd. NE
Atlanta, GA 30333
website: www.cdc.gov

The CDC is the United States' leading health protection agency. Numerous publications about lead contamination can be found on its website, including articles about the hazards of lead paint, lead in drinking water, lead in soil, and lead in children's toys.

Coalition to Prevent Lead Poisoning
1150 University Ave.
Rochester, NY 14607
website: http://theleadcoalition.org

The Coalition to Prevent Lead Poisoning is an education and advocacy organization that is dedicated to eliminating childhood lead poisoning and other environmental home health hazards. Its website offers a wide variety of publications on the causes of lead contamination, children who have been poisoned by lead, how lead poisoning can be prevented, and other topics.

Earthjustice
50 California St., Suite 500
San Francisco, CA 94111
website: https://earthjustice.org

As the United States' largest nonprofit environmental law organization, Earthjustice puts the law to use to fight for and protect people's health and the environment. Its website search engine produces numerous publications about lead contamination and other lead-related issues.

Lead Poisoning, *U.S. News & World Report*
website: www.usnews.com/topics/subjects/lead_poisoning

This is an excellent collection of articles that cover topics such as widespread lead contamination on US Army bases, schools testing students for blood lead levels, deaths related to lead exposure, lead contamination cleanup efforts, safety dangers in older houses, and many others.

National Institute of Environmental Health Sciences (NIEHS)
PO Box 12233, Mail Drop K3-16
Research Triangle Park, NC 27709
website: www.niehs.nih.gov

A member of the National Institutes of Health, the NIEHS conducts research into the effects of the environment on human health. Its website features a number of publications about lead, how people are exposed to it, and the many types of health problems it can cause.

US Department of Housing and Urban Development (HUD)
Healthy Homes and Lead Hazard Control
451 Seventh St. SW, Rm. B-133
Washington, DC 20410
website: www.hud.gov

HUD is an agency of the federal government that seeks to expand home ownership, increase access to affordable housing, strengthen communities through economic development, and fight housing discrimination. Its website offers publications on sources of lead contamination, lead paint in homes, the effects of lead exposure, lead poisoning, and other related topics.

US Environmental Protection Agency (EPA)
401 M St. SW
Washington, DC 20460
website: www.epa.gov

The EPA's mission is to protect human health and the environment. Its website has a separate section on lead that offers a wealth of information about how lead contaminates the soil, air, and water; the dangers of careless removal of lead paint; how lead exposure affects children and the harm it can cause; and many other related topics.

FOR FURTHER RESEARCH

Books

Bridge Magazine staff, *Poison on Tap*. Traverse City, MI: Mission Point, 2016.

Anna Clark, *The Poisoned City: Flint's Water and the American Urban Tragedy*. New York: Metropolitan, 2018.

Mona Hanna-Attisha, *What the Eyes Don't See*. New York: One World, 2018.

Gerald Markowitz and David Rosner, *Lead Wars*. Berkeley: University of California Press, 2013.

Internet Sources

Rae Ellen Bichell, "Childhood Exposure to Lead Can Blunt IQ for Decades, Study Suggests," NPR, March 28, 2017. www.npr.org.

Angus Chen, "Lead Dust from Firearms Can Pose a Silent Health Risk," NPR, May 10, 2017. www.npr.org.

Brenda Goodman et al., "There's Lead in That?!," WebMD, September 6, 2017. www.webmd.com.

J. David Goodman et al., "Tests Showed Children Were Exposed to Lead. The Official Response: Challenge the Tests," *New York Times*, November 18, 2018. www.nytimes.com.

Michael Hawthorne and Cecilia Reyes, "Brain-Damaging Lead Found in Tap Water in Hundreds of Homes Tested Across Chicago, Results Show," *Chicago Tribune*, April 12, 2018. www.chicagotribune.com.

Terrence McCoy, "Washington's Worst Case of Lead Poisoning in Decades Happened in a Home Sanctioned by Housing Officials," *Washington Post*, January 30, 2017. www.washingtonpost.com.

M.B. Pell and Joshua Schneyer, "Special Report: Thousands of U.S. Areas Afflicted with Lead Poisoning Beyond Flint's," Reuters, December 19, 2016. www.reuters.com.

Eliza Shapiro, "More than 1,100 School Faucets Still Have Lead, City Says," *New York Times*, September 11, 2018. www.nytimes.com.

INDEX

Note: Boldface page numbers indicate illustrations.

Aloshen, Debbie, 54
American Public Health Association, 68
American Water Works Association, 44–45
attention deficit hyperactivity disorder (ADHD), 28

baby food, lead contamination of, 17
Baker, Bianca, 45
Baraka, Ras, 21
Barnes, Miki, 48
Bellinger, David, 50–53
Benfer, Emily A., 49, 50
Bhambhani, Kanta J., 25–26
blood-brain barrier, 24
blood lead levels
 decline of, in children, 22, 36, **38**
 in Detroit children, 15–16
 reference level for, 26–27
Bonaparte, Mikaila, 43–44
brain
 impact of lead on, 28
  developmental disabilities and, 33–35
  intelligence and, 31–33
 vulnerability to lead exposure, 25
Brooks, Larry, 16
Brown, Darlena, 34–35
Brown, Edward, 40
Brown, John Cale "JC," Jr., 34–35

calcium, 23–24
Centers for Disease Control and Prevention (CDC), 26–27, 36, 37, 44, 68
 on flushing home plumbing systems, 56
Chicago Tribune (newspaper), 45
children
 blood lead levels in
  decline in, 22, **38**
  prevalence of elevated levels, 36
  reference level for, 26–27
  testing for, **55**
 health issues linked to lead in, 28
 lead dust as primary source of lead poisoning in, 12–13
 vulnerability of, to lead exposure, 24–26
chromium, 23

Cleveland, OH, program to address lead exposure in, 53–54
Coalition to Prevent Lead Poisoning, 68
Collins, Michael, 11
Consumer Product Safety Commission (CPSC), 20
crime, connection between lead and, 47
Currie, Janet, 59–60
Curtis, Jana, 18

Department of Housing and Urban Development, US (HUD), 42, 69–70
Detroit Health Department, 15–16
developmental disabilities, 33–35
Drum, Kevin, 47
dyslexia, 28

Earthjustice, 69
Edwards, Marc, 36
Environmental Defense Fund, 17
Environmental Protection Agency, US (EPA), 11, 20, 22, 47, 70

Federal Aviation Administration (FAA), 46
fertility, effects of lead on, 26
Filippelli, Gabriel, 61
Flint (MI)/Flint water crisis, 6–7, **8,** 19–21, 54–55, 62
  gift of new water systems for schools in, 52
  impact on children's reading proficiency, 32–33
  low-income housing in, **41**
  miscarriage rates and, 29–30
  poverty and, 40–41
Food and Drug Administration, US, 45

gasoline
  aviation (avgas), 46–48
  lead in, 7, 18
Gearing, Mary, 23, 24
Grossman, Daniel, 29–30

Haak, Liz, 14
Hanna-Attisha, Mona, 6, 24, 32
Harvard Environmental Law Review, 49
health risks of lead
  in adults, 30
  in children, 28
  developmental, 33–35
Heiger-Bernays, Wendy, 11
Higgins, John, 59, 60–61
housing demolition, risk of lead dust from, 14–16
Hughes, Karla, 59

Indiana University—Purdue University Indianapolis (IUPUI), 61
Irwin, Tom, 57, 58

Jacobs, David, 10–11
Januta, Andrea, 58

Katner, Adrienne, 56
Ketterer, Michael, 16
Khaldun, Joneigh, 16

Landrigan, Philip, 33, 50–53
Lanphear, Bruce P., 24–25, 30, 32, 50
lead
   dangers of first recognized, 7
   effects on body, 23–24
   effects on fertility, 26
   need for identifying sources of, 51–52
lead contamination
   from aviation gasoline, 46–48
   of baby food, 17
   of drinking water, **8**
      checking for, **60**
      EPA action level for, 43
      in Flint, MI, 6–7, 19–21, 54–55, 62
      in Newark, NJ, 21
      public awareness of, 8–9
      gap in data on extent of, 37
      lack of nationwide effort to address, 49
   in NY public housing, 42–44
   poverty and risk of, 40–42
   of soil, 16–18
      as source of household contamination, 61
   in South Bend, IN, 40
   in St. Joseph, MO, 39–40
   of toys, 20
   See also prevention programs
lead-crime hypothesis, 47
lead pipes, **19**
   prevalence of, 44–45
Lead Poisoning, *U.S. News & World Report* (website), 69
Lead Renovation, Repair and Painting Rule (RRP Rule), 11
learning disabilities, 28
legacy lead, 45
Levy, Daniel, 28
Lopez, Derrick, 52
Lotas, Lynn, 54
Luster, Heavenz, 27–28

Mallya, Giridhar, 54
Markel, Howard, 27, 40–42
McCush, Gerald, 39
McMullen, Tolanda, 42
McNeill, Fiona E., 7
metals, human health and, 23

Michigan, efforts to address lead exposure in, 54–57
Midgley, Thomas, Jr., 7
Mignery, Lauranda, 39–40
Musk, Elon, 52

National Institute of Environmental Health Sciences (NIEHS), 69
Natural Resources Defense Council, 21
Neltner, Tom, 17
New Hampshire, efforts to address lead exposure in, 57–58
New York City Housing Authority (Nycha), 42–44

Obama, Barack, 6
Olson, Erik, 21, 56–57
orthophosphate, 20

paint, lead-based, 7
  lead dust and, 12–14
  prevalence of, 10–11
  removal of, **12**
Partners in Health Lead Screening Program (Cleveland, OH), 53–54, **55**
Pell, M.B., 37, 38
Philadelphia
  children with elevated blood lead levels in, 39
  industrial lead contamination in, 18
  lead contamination in soil in, 16–17
poverty, risk of lead contamination and, 40–42
pregnancy, dangers of lead exposure during, 28–31
prevention programs
  in Cleveland, OH, 53–54, **55**
  essential phases of, 51–53
  in Michigan, 54–57
  on military bases, 58–59
  in New Hampshire, 57–58
  in New Jersey, 59–61
Princeton University, 59–61

Robinson, Loren, 39
Roper, Cyndi, 55
Ruderman, Wendy, 17
Rumpler, John, 43

Schneider, Jay, 35
Schneyer, Joshua, 37, 38, 58
Schulte, Elaine, 9
Sherwin-Williams, 10
Slaughter, Freddie Mae, 13
Slusky, David, 29–30
survey, on awareness of lead contamination, 8–9

tetraethyl lead, 7
toys, lead in, 20

Urban Tap Water and Human Health project (Trenton, NJ), 59–61

Vitruvius, Marcus, 7

Wargovich, Maria, 13
water
  lead contamination of
    EPA action level for, 43
    gap in data on extent of, 37
    lead pipes and, 44–45
    in Newark, NJ, 21
    public awareness of, 8–9
    in schools, 43
    See also Flint (MI)/Flint water crisis
Water Quality Association, 8–9

zinc, 23

PICTURE CREDITS

Cover: MoMorad/iStockphoto.com

8: Ryan Garza/Zuma Press/Newscom
12: Christian Delbert/Shutterstock.com
15: ungvar/Shutterstock.com
19: micmacpics/Shutterstock.com
25: Duplass/Shutterstock.com
29: Odua Images/Shutterstock.com
32: Levranii/Shutterstock.com
38: Maury Aaseng
41: TennesseePhotographer/iStockphoto.com
46: dragunov/Shutterstock.com
51: Terentieva Yulia/Shutterstock.com
55: Degimages/Shutterstock.com
60: dusanpetkovic/Shutterstock.com

ABOUT THE AUTHOR

Peggy J. Parks has written dozens of educational books on a wide variety of topics for children, teens, and young adults. She holds a bachelor's degree from Aquinas College in Grand Rapids, Michigan, where she graduated magna cum laude. Parks lives in Muskegon, Michigan, a town she says inspires her writing because of its location on the shores of beautiful Lake Michigan.